Plasticity in Nerve Cell Function

Monographs of the Physiological Society

43. Dwain L. Eckberg and Peter Slight, *Human Baroreflexes in Health Disease,* 1992

44. Christopher L-H. Huang, *Intramembrane Charge Movements in Striated Muscle,* 1993

45. Robert Porter and Roger Lemon, *Corticospinal Function and Voluntary Movement,* 1993

46. M. de Burgh Daly, *Peripheral Arterial Chemoreceptors and Respiratory-Cardiovascular Integration,* 1997

47. Platon Kostyuk, *Plasticity in nerve cell function,* 1998

Plasticity in Nerve Cell Function

Platon Kostyuk
Bogomoletz Institute of Physiology
Kiev, Ukraine

CLARENDON PRESS • OXFORD
1998

Oxford University Press, Great Clarendon Street, Oxford OX2 6DP

Oxford New York
Athens Auckland Bangkok Bogota Bombay Buenos Aires Calcutta
Cape Town Chennai Dar es Salaam Delhi Florence Hong Kong Istanbul
Karachi Kuala Lumpur Madrid Melbourne Mexico City Mumbai
Nairobi Paris São Paolo Singapore Taipei Tokyo Toronto Warsaw

and associated companies in
Berlin Ibadan

Oxford is a trade mark of Oxford University Press

Published in the United States
by Oxford University Press, Inc., New York

A catalogue record for this book is available from the British Library

Library of Congress Cataloging in Publication Data
(Data available)

ISBN 0 19 852418 8

Typeset by Footnote Graphics, Warminster, Wilts

Printed in Great Britain by
Biddles Ltd, Guildford & King's Lynn

Preface

The specific functional feature of the nervous system that distinguishes it from all other systems in living organisms is its ability to accept an immense flow of external stimuli, transform them into neuronal messages, and analyse, store, and compare them with previous inputs. The nervous system changes the functioning of all other systems through the results of this processing, providing the organism with appropriate reactions that enable its survival in its interactions with the external environment. To fulfil this extremely complicated task, the nervous system has to be capable of matching its function with the changes which occur in the organism during its life span—beginning from the embryonic period and extending into ageing. At the same time it must adjust its function to more short-lived changes such as wakefulness and sleep, relaxation and stress; it has to maintain its activity as far as possible during pathological conditions to give the organism a chance to survive. The nervous system can meet all these demands due to the extreme flexibility of the structural and functional properties of its elements—both neuronal and glial—which can change their form, molecular organization, and interconnections over different time scales—from minutes to days and months. This unique feature of the nervous system can be most properly described as *plasticity* in a broad sense, as compared with the frequent use of this term to describe only prolonged changes in the effectiveness of synaptic transmission. The present monograph seeks to analyse plastic changes in the functioning of neuronal and glial elements from such a broad perspective. The available data have led to the conclusion that in all forms of plastic changes in the functioning of the nervous system there are common basic mechanisms, changes in the level of free Ca^{2+} ions in the cytosol being one of them. In conjunction with other more specific molecular mechanisms, these 'calcium signals' participate in an extremely complicated intracellular machinery that is capable of controlling all the structural and functional properties of the nervous system during its whole life span and during the possible demands that it may meet in-between. The key role of Ca^{2+} ions in nerve cell function has been of significant interest in neuroscience for many years, and it has already been reviewed in another book published by Oxford University Press (Kostyuk 1992). However, the progress in this field has been so rapid that it justifies further consideration of the problem from a different point of view.

The author is extremely grateful to the Bogomoletz Institute of Physiology of the National Academy of Sciences of the Ukraine where he has worked for almost forty years and where he has enjoyed a high scientific spirit, all possible help from his collaborators, and excellent technical facilities.

Kiev P. K.
September 1997

Contents

Previous volumes in this series

Published by Edward Arnold

1. H. Barcroft and H. J. C. Swan, *Sympathetic Control of Human Blood Vessels*, 1953
2. A. C. Burton and O. G. Edholm, *Man in a Cold Environment*, 1955
3. G. W. Harris, *Neural Control of the Pituitary Gland*, 1955
4. A. H. James, *Physiology of Gastric Digestion*, 1957
5. B. Delisle Burns, *The Mammalian Cerebral Cortex*, 1958
6. G. S. Brindley, *Physiology of the Retina and Visual Pathway*, 1960 (2nd edition 1970)
7. D. A. McDonald, *Blood Flow in Arteries*, 1960
8. A. S. V. Burgen and N. G. Emmelin, *Physiology of the Salivary Glands*, 1961
9. Audrey U. Smith, *Biological Effects of Freezing and Super-cooling*, 1961
10. W. J. O'Connor, *Renal Function*, 1962
11. R. A. Gregory, *Secretory Mechanisms of the Gastro-Intestinal Tract*, 1962
12. C. A. Keele and Desiree Armstrong, *Substances Producing Pain and Itch*, 1964
13. R. Whittam, *Transport and Diffusion in Red Blood Cells*, 1964
14. J. Grayson and D. Mendel, *Physiology of the Splanchnic Circulation*, 1965
15. B. T. Donovan and J. J. van der Werff ten Bosch, *Physiology of* Puberty, 1965
16. I. de Burgh Daly and Catherine Hebb, *Pulmonary and Bronchial Vascular Systems*, 1966
17. I. C. Whitfield, *The Auditory Pathway*, 1967
18. L. E. Mount, *The Climatic Physiology of the Pig*, 1968
19. J. I. Hubbard, R Llinàs, and D. Quastel, *Electrophysiological Analysis of Synaptic Transmission*, 1969
20. S. E. Dicker, *Mechanisms of Urine Concentration and Dilution in Mammals*, 1970
21. G. Kahlson and Elsa Rosengren, *Biogenesis and Physiology of Histamine*, 1971

22. A. T. Cowie and J. S. Tindal, *The Physiology of Lactation*, 1971
23. Peter B. C. Matthews, *Mammalian Muscle Receptors and their Central Actions*, 1972
24. C. R. House, *Water Transport in Cells and Tissues*, 1974
25. P. P. Newman, *Visceral Afferent Functions of the Nervous System*, 1974
28. M. J. Purves, *The Physiology of the Cerebral Circulation*, 1972

Published by Cambridge University Press

29. D. McK. Kerslake, *The Stress of Hot Environments*, 1972
30. M. R. Bennett, *Autonomic Neuromuscular Transmission*, 1972
31. A. G. Macdonald, *Physiological Aspects of Deep Sea Biology*, 1975
32. M. Peaker and J. L. Linzell, *Salt Glands in Birds and Reptiles*, 1975
33. J. A. Barrowman, *Physiology of the Gastro-intestinal Lymphatic System*, 1978
35. J. T. Fitzsimmons, *The Physiology of Thirst and Sodium Appetite*, 1979
39. R. J. Linden and C. T. Kappagoda, *Atrial Receptors*, 1982
40. R. Elsner and B. Gooden, *Diving and Asphyxia*, 1983

Published by Academic Press

34. C. G. Phillips and R. Porter, *Corticospinal Neurones, Their Role in Movements*, 1977
36. O. H. Petersen, *The Electrophysiology of Gland Cells*, 1980
37. W. R. Keatinge and M. Clare Harman, *Local Mechanisms Controlling Blood Vessels*, 1980
38. H. Hensel, *Thermoreception and Temperature Regulation*, 1981
41. R. C. Woledge, N. Curtin, and E. Homsher, *Energetic Aspects of Muscle Contraction*, 1984
42. J. R. Henderson, *'Mémoir sur le Pancreas', by Claude Bernard* (Translation), 1985

All these volumes are now out of print.

1

Formation of neuronal networks

GENERAL FEATURES

The functioning of the nervous system begins with the formation of the neuronal network from undifferentiated neuronal precursors. This process is of extreme complexity and includes many interconnected steps during which important changes occur in the structure and functional properties of the involved elements. Cellular and molecular mechanisms of these changes have been investigated step by step both in *in vivo* experiments and in experiments in model systems—cell cultures obtained from neuronal elements of different developmental stages. Somewhat schematically the formation of neuronal networks can be separated into the following stages: movement of the precursor cells to the places of their final location, initiation of neurite outgrowth, targeting of their direction, establishment of contacts with the targets, formation of synaptic structures, and elimination of elements which did not find their purpose. To some extent this process can be reproduced in case of injury and regeneration of brain structures, when the axons of the surviving cells again have to find their way to their targets and form functional connections.

ORIGIN AND MIGRATION OF NEURONAL PRECURSORS

Neural stem cells are competent to generate neurons, astrocytes, and oligodendrocytes. It is not yet clear to what extent these fates are specified intrinsically or influenced by environmental factors. It is possible that neural stem cells are intrinsically programmed to generate progeny of all these fates randomly, and environment selects among them and regulates further development; another possibility is that neural stem cells are programmed to generate just one of these fates, and environmental factors direct them into other lineage pathways. Some indications in favour of the second possibility have been recently obtained on mice embryonic cerebral cortex. Here the early cortical stem cells are neuronal and quite heterogeneous in the number of neurons that they generate. In low fibroblast growth factor (FGF2) concentrations most of them maintain this specification, generating solely neuronal progeny. Oligodendroglial production within these clones is stimulated by a higher, threshold level of FGF2, and astrocyte production requires additional environmental glia-inducing factors. Correspondingly, *in vivo* most cortical neurons are born before glia (Qian *et al.* 1997).

During the embryonic development of the future nervous system the post-mitotic neuronal precursors generated near the ventricular surface of the neuronal tube have to migrate substantial distances to reach their final destination. This obviously requires a well-organized migration pattern based on interaction between the migrating cell and the adhesive molecules and structural elements in its environment. Glial fibres may play such a guiding role in migration as has been directly shown in the embryonic cerebral cortex, cell-surface glycoproteins being involved in the identification of the migrating neurons and their commitment to specific regions (cf. Mione and Parnavelas 1994). The same has been shown for migrating Purkinje neurons in the cerebellum, guided by radial glial processes through cell adhesion (Yuasa *et al.* 1996). Some specific processes have to be triggered in the migrating cell itself, causing changes in cell shape and its transplantation. It has been shown that even at this early developmental stage the intracellular signal responsible for these events might be carried by Ca^{2+} ions. Thus, in developing cerebellar cortex the migration of granule cells to their mature position starts only after expression of N-type Ca^{2+} channels in their membrane. Their selective blockade by ω-conotoxin curtailed such movement, while inhibition of L- and T-type channels had no such effect. Obviously, influx of Ca^{2+} at specific cellular sites must be critical for directed migration; such influx through NMDA-channels could also support movement (Komuro and Rakic 1992, 1993).

NEURITE INDUCTION

Induction of the outgrowth of neurites is the next crucial step, which is the most obvious sign of the beginning of neuronal differentiation.

Under model conditions, for example cell cultures, it can be triggered by several external influences, including nerve-growth factors (NGF), and therefore can be extensively analysed.

The beginning of this process is again related to changes in intracellular Ca^{2+} homeostasis in the form of elevation of the resting level of $[Ca^{2+}]_i$ (intracellular Ca^{2+}) and the appearance of calcium transients and waves. These events have been traced in several systems—amphibian and mammalian neurons in culture, neuroblastoma and pheochromocytoma cell lines, etc. At the very beginning of differentiation transient elevations of $[Ca^{2+}]_i$ always appear. This spontaneous process requires Ca^{2+} influx through both low- and high-voltage-activated (LVA and HVA) Ca^{2+} channels; the first might be of special importance as they are found to be expressed even in non-differentiated cells, and their density increases at the beginning of differentiation (Veselovsky *et al.* 1984; Vyatchenko-Karpinskii *et al.* 1995*a*). In cultured chick dorsal root ganglion (DRG) precursor neurons (taken from embryonic day 6) functionally undifferentiated cells (during the first 10 h in culture) also expressed only LVA Ca^{2+} currents; HVA Ca^{2+} and Na^+ currents appeared delayed after more than 10 h in culture (Gottmann *et al.* 1991).

Figure 1.1 presents the characteristics of LVA Ca^{2+} currents recorded from a neuroblastoma cell at the beginning of its differentiation induced by increasing the pH of the culture medium; these currents were the only type of Ca^{2+} channel activity recorded at this stage.

As activation of LVA Ca^{2+} channels takes place even at membrane potentials close to its resting level, it may easily trigger low-threshold Ca^{2+} transients. Following influx of Ca^{2+} ions from the

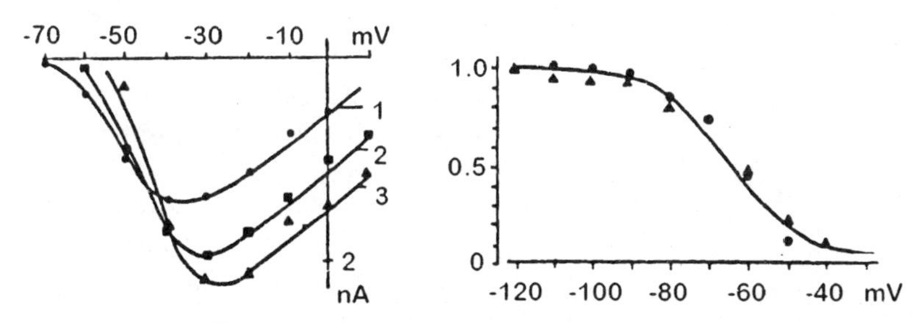

FIG 1.1 LVA Ca^{2+} currents expressed in mouse neuroblastoma cells at the beginning of induced differentiation. (A): current–voltage characteristics obtained with external Ca^{2+} concentrations 5 (1), 15 (2), and 40 (3) mM; (B): steady-state inactivation curve (from Veselovsky *et al.* 1984).

extracellular space, Ca^{2+}-induced Ca^{2+} release from intracellular stores can substantially amplify the intracellular transients; it seems that such release is most effective at the early stages of neuronal development and declines during subsequent stages. These processes may initiate two distinct types of spontaneous elevation of $[Ca^{2+}]_i$—fast spikes and more slowly developing waves, which can be differently expressed in different neurons from the same brain structure (cf. Spitzer *et al.* 1992, 1995; Spitzer 1991, 1994). Spikes are usually observed in neurons before neurite expansion, and their frequency decreases with time in culture, while the frequency of waves appears to be constant, and they propagate into the growth cones of growing neurites (Gu and Spitzer 1997). The increased expression of membrane ion-channels at the beginning of differentiation is in some way related to the activity of protein kinase C (PKC), as its down-regulation by selective inhibitors reduces the density of channels (Reuter *et al.* 1992).

When the cells start to differentiate, reciprocal changes in the densities of Ca^{2+} and other types of ion channel (Na^+) may occur. If differentiation is progressing, the density of Ca^{2+} channels start to decrease, while that of Na^+ channels progressively increases; inhibition of differentiation and return to proliferation induces opposite changes. A convenient method to reveal this correlation is the pH change of the culture medium—an increase in pH to 7.8–8.2 induced differentiation, while a decrease below 7.4 stimulated return to proliferation (Veselovsky and Fomina 1986). Figure 1.2. illustrates the described reciprocal changes in the densities of both currents and the corresponding correlation.

It should be taken into account, that the triggering effect of intracellular Ca^{2+} on neurite outgrowth has a definite concentration optimum—excessive elevations of $[Ca^{2+}]_i$ have a depressive effect. Measurements on developing rat sensory neurons have shown the presence of a quite narrow concentration window; maximal outgrowth was observed at 35 nM $[Ca^{2+}]_i$; different neurons again could have different set-points for starting the outgrowth or survival (Al-Mohanna *et al.* 1992). Because of this high sensitivity of the triggering mechanisms, they can be effectively manipulated by even small changes in the cellular environment affecting the influx of Ca^{2+} ions. Thus, addition of low concentrations of Ca-channel blockers has been shown to stimulate the differentiation of murine neuroblastoma cells and the increase in density of LVA Ca^{2+} channels in their membrane, while high concentrations suppressed the viability

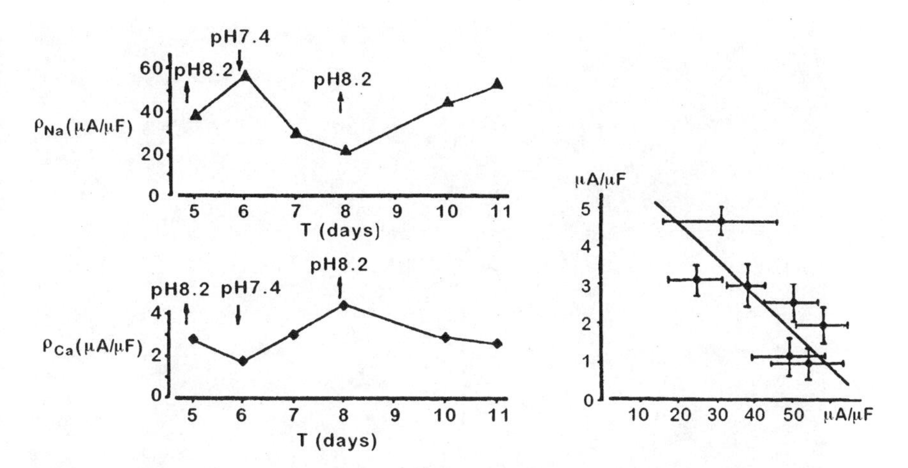

FIG 1.2 Reciprocal changes in the densities of LVA Ca^{2+} and TTX-sensitive Na^{+} currents in mouse neuroblastoma cells during progressing differentiation or return to proliferation triggered by pH changes of the culture medium. (A): mean current densities, (B): correlation between densities of Ca^{2+} (abscissa) and Na^{+} (ordinate) currents described by linear regression equation (from Veselovsky and Fomina 1986).

of cells and induced retraction of their processes. Obviously, even resting leakage of Ca^{2+} into the cell by spontaneously active voltage-operated Ca^{2+} channels (VOCC) may exceed the above mentioned optimal window of intracellular free calcium; this may be the reason why culturing of cells in the presence of a low concentration of Ca-channel blockers may stimulate differentiation (Vyatchenko-Karpinskii *et al.* 1995*b*; Starikova *et al.* 1997). Figure 1.3 illustrates the effective induction of differentiation in our experiments on PC12 pheochromocytoma cells cultured in a medium with addition of nifedipine, most effective at 5 μM concentration, and Fig. 1.4—statistical data about morphological changes in the investigated cells—indicates initial suppression of proliferation already occurring at the 3rd day in culture (A) and steep increase in the outgrowth of neurites (B) starting at the 5th day of culturing. A parallel measurement of the $[Ca^{2+}]_i$ level in the same cells (C) indicated that addition of 2.5 and 5 μM nifedipine induced a substantial *decrease* of this level to values of about 50 nM, most prominent during suppression of proliferation (3rd day of culturing). This level is close to the above mentioned level of $[Ca^{2+}]_i$ necessary for induction of differentiation in cultured sensory neurons. The induction of neurite outgrowth, which started 2 d later, occurred at an already increasing

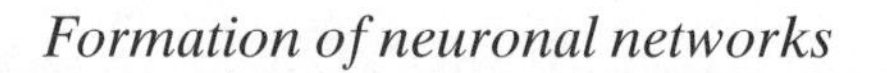

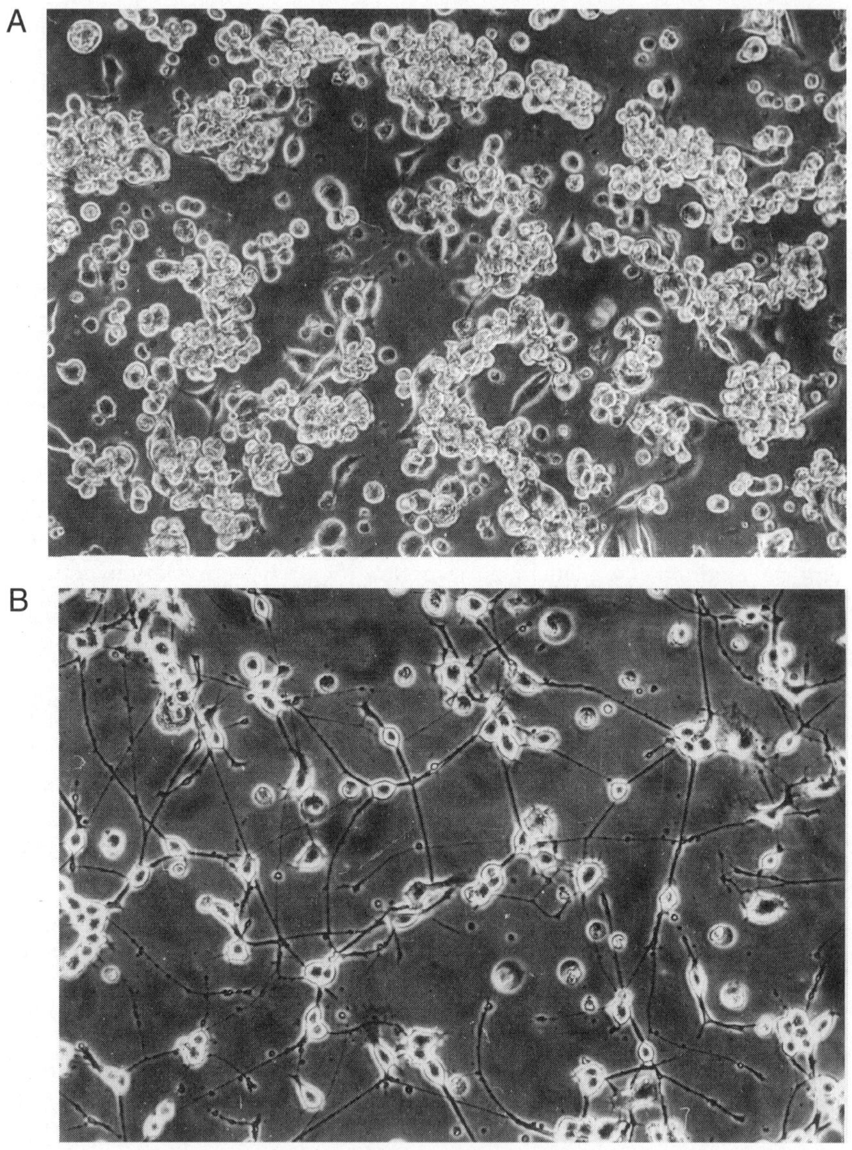

FIG 1.3 Induction of differentiation in PC12 pheochromocytoma cells by culturing them in a medium containing 5 μM nifedipine. (A): control cells, (B): after 4 d culturing in the nifedipine-containing medium (Starikova *et al.* 1998).

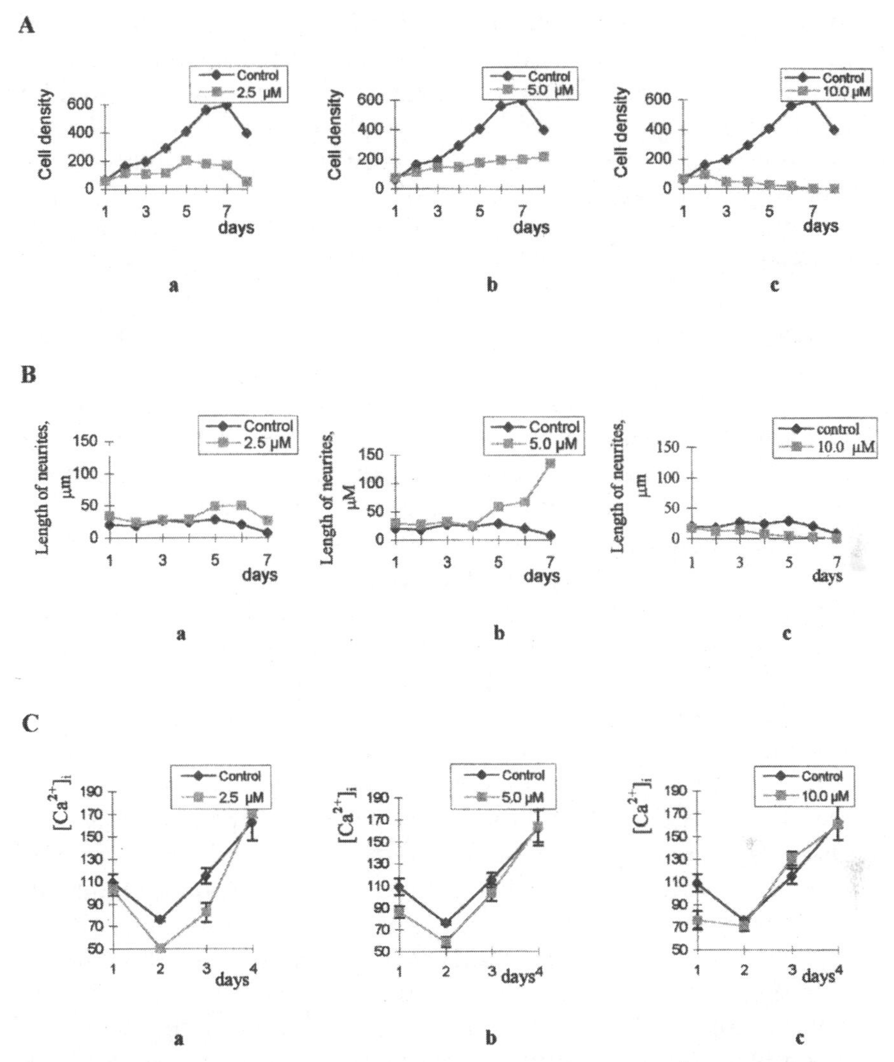

FIG 1.4 Changes in morphological characteristics and $[Ca^{2+}]_i$ level of PC12 cells cultured in the presence of 2.5 (a), 5 (b), and 10 μM (c) nifedipine. (A): changes in cell density, (B): changes in the length of neurites, (C): changes in $[Ca^{2+}]_i$ (Starikova *et al.* 1998).

level of $[Ca^{2+}]_i$; this may indicate that different optimal levels of intracellular Ca^{2+} may be necessary for suppression of proliferation and for induction of neurite outgrowth.

The mechanisms of such down-regulatory effect of verapamil or nifedipine on $[Ca^{2+}]_i$ is not quite clear; probably it is due to suppression of spontaneous activation of L-type Ca^{2+} channels already present in the cellular membrane. Higher concentrations of Ca^{2+}-channel blockers induced a damaging effect manifested by a progressive increase in $[Ca^{2+}]_i$ and neurite destruction. It should be kept in mind that an organic Ca^{2+}-channel blocker like verapamil can by itself induce unspecific changes in membrane permeability; it has been shown Hübschle *et al.* (1997) on rat-brain RNA injected oocytes that verapamil can increase the membrane leakage permeability for K^+ and Cl^- ions which might be responsible for such destructive effects.

Measurements of the dependence of neurite outgrowth on the intracellular level of Ca^{2+} were made also on cultured cerebellar granule cells. They also demonstrated a bell-shaped dependence with a peak between 37 and 108 nM $[Ca^{2+}]_i$. However, it should be mentioned that the situation was different in some other experiments: in N1E-115 neuroblastoma cells the outgrowth was found to decrease monotonically with elevation of intracellular Ca^{2+} (Zimprich *et al.* 1994). The inhibitory effect of elevated intracellular Ca^{2+} can be dependent on the activation of Ca-dependent proteinases (calpains) affecting cytoskeletal proteins. It has been shown on isolated developing hippocampal pyramidal neurons that application of a Ca^{2+} ionophore suppresses neurite outgrowth and induces retraction of dendritic processes; administration of a calpain inhibitor to the culture medium completely blocked this effect of the ionophore, although the inhibitor was ineffective by itself (Song *et al.* 1994). A similar inhibitory effect on the outgrowth of neurites is exerted by the anti-tumour substance suramin (polysulphonated naphthylurea)—presumably also by creating excessive Ca^{2+} influx because in Ca^{2+}-free extracellular medium the outgrowth could be restored; nimodipine mimicked the protective role of Ca^{2+}-free solution (Sun *et al.* 1995). Ca^{2+} release from intracellular stores may be important in the determination of this level (cf. review by Gill *et al.* 1996). Thus, depletion of intracellular Ca^{2+} stores in cultured developing *Xenopus* neurons at early stages affected their differentiation in a manner similar to the prevention of Ca^{2+} influx (Holliday *et al.* 1991). At early stages of development (in cultured embryonic amphibian neurons) spontaneous transient intracellular calcium elevations were often observed which may also contribute to differentiation (Holliday and Spitzer 1990).

The induction of differentiation by these intracellular signals is mediated through corresponding changes in genomic expression. This was anticipated quite a long time ago on the basis of experiments with induction of neurite outgrowth in neuroblastoma cells by injection of db-cAMP (Lieberman and Sachs 1978). Ca^{2+}-dependent stimulation of phosphorylation of some proteins is a necessary step in this process (Mehta *et al.* 1993). More recently it has been shown that intracellular messengers cause rapid activation of tyrosine kinases which include non-receptor tyrosine kinase (Src). Protein tyrosine phosphorylation results in formation of linker proteins and subsequent activation of GTP-binding proteins (Ras) and mitogen-activated protein (MAP) kinases followed by induction of immediate early genes (IEG). A large number of distinct IEGs have been identified in neuronal elements, and it is likely that many IEGs remain to be identified. Several IEGs, including the well known *c-fos* proto-oncogene, encode transcription factors that regulate expression of late-response genes which in turn encode protein synthesis necessary for neuronal growth and differentiation. There are at least two distinct DNA motifs within the regulatory region of *c-fos* that are critical for calcium activation of the *c-fos* transcription—the CRE (cAMP response element) and SRE (serum response element). CRE after phosphorylation by different kinases on Ser^{133} and binding of transcriptional co-activator proteins may confer induction of an otherwise non-responsive gene. In addition to the action of Ca^{2+}-dependent protein kinases, the phosphorylation state of the element can be modulated by Ca^{2+}-dependent protein phosphatases. Therefore spatially distinct Ca^{2+} signals to the nucleus may influence the activation of transcription factor complexes in unique ways. SRE may be also important mediators of Ca^{2+}-sensitive *c-fos* transcription, mediating the effect of NGF and other growth factors (cf. recent review by Ginty 1997).

All these mechanisms and the induction of neurite outgrowth are inhibited by the expression of dominant negative forms of both Src and Ras (Rusanescu *et al.* 1995). It should be mentioned that some data do not correspond to this general scheme giving a prominent role to Ca^{2+}-dependent protein phosphorylation in triggering neuronal differentiation. Thus, it has been shown in PC12 cells that okadaic acid (a protein phosphatase inhibitor) which may support phosphorylation inhibits NGF-directed neurite outgrowth (Chiou and Westhead 1992).

A natural mechanism which can limit the elevations of intracellular Ca^{2+} during later stages of differentiation, when they may become excessive, is the functional expression of potassium currents in a transcription-dependent manner. The resulting changes promote the shortening of action potentials and the reduction of Ca^{2+} influx, although calcium channels are still present (cf. Spitzer 1991).

An important question which only recently became an object of experimental investigation is the determination of pathways by which cytoplasmic Ca^{2+} signals may reach the intranuclear structures. Usually it is accepted that the intranuclear space is easily accessible to cytosolic factors, including Ca^{2+} ions, by diffusion due to the presence of large pores in the nuclear membrane. However, recently it has been shown that the nuclear envelop in fact forms a calcium store which can effectively accumulate Ca^{2+} from the cytosol and is formed probably by the nuclear membrane itself and the adjacent membrane of the endoplasmic reticulum. Most important is the finding that this store can rapidly inject Ca^{2+} into the nucleoplasm in response to ligands that activate Ca^{2+}-release channels (IP_3, cADPribose) and in this way greatly accelerate and amplify intranuclear calcium signalling (Gerasimenko *et al.* 1995, 1996*a*). In correlation with these data is the finding that IP_3 can bc produced inside the nucleus and act on receptors located at the inner nuclear membrane (Humbert *et al.* 1996).

Activation of corresponding receptors by NGF is an obligatory cofactor in the induction of neurite outgrowth; however, NGF alone is less effective and has to be combined with other factors triggering intracellular signals like membrane depolarization and corresponding changes in intracellular Ca^{2+} (Solem *et al.* 1995). On the other hand, although depolarization alone preserves preexisting neurites, unlike NGF, it does not itself promote neurite elongation (Teng and Greene 1993). A synergistic effect on neurite outgrowth is also observed in PC12 cells between NGF and dibutyryl cAMP. To evaluate the possible mechanisms of such interaction, the cells were treated with both factors for 2 d, and then the effects on neurite outgrowth of Ca^{2+} influx or Ca^{2+} mobilization from intracellular stores were tested. It was found that both influences enhanced Ca^{2+} accumulation by non-mitochondrial (thapsigargin-sensitive) Ca^{2+} pools. Depletion of intracellular Ca^{2+} stores by thapsigargin significantly inhibited the stimulating effect of dbcAMP or of dbCAMP+NGF, but did not affect NGF-stimulated outgrowth. Thus both factors seem to involve intracellular Ca^{2+} although through different pathways (Huang *et al.* 1996).

The participation of Ca^{2+}/calmodulin-dependent protein kinase II (CaMKII) in NGF-induced cell differentiation has also to be taken into account. In experiments on PC12 pheochromocytoma cells with over-expressed CaMKII altered cellular growth and adhesion properties were observed, including increased cell-to-substrate adhesion, decreased cell-to-cell adhesion and inhibited neurite elongation during NGF-induced differentiation . The changes could be reversed by kinase inhibitor KN-62 (Masse and Kelly 1997). The mechanisms underlying such effects have to be analysed; they may depend on the dynamic balance between Ca^{2+}/CaM-dependent protein kinase and phosphatase activities and probably also involve regulation of gene expression. Other observations have shown that Ca^{2+}/CaM-dependent protein phosphatase (calcineurin) also participate in neurite outgrowth (Chang *et al.* 1995).

An interesting applied question in this respect is the interaction of NGF and elevated intracellular Ca^{2+} in the background of acute ethanol treatment. Ethanol neurotoxicity is extremely dangerous at early developmental stages, resulting in substantial loss of neurons. It has been shown on rat septal neurons cultured on the day of birth (PO) that NGF can ameliorate this neurotoxic effect by acting on ethanol-induced changes of $[Ca^{2+}]_i$. Ethanol at behaviourally relevant levels caused a rapid damaging increase of $[Ca^{2+}]_i$, while NGF exerted a protective effect via lowering $[Ca^{2+}]_i$ (Webb *et al.* 1996).

Basic fibroblast growth factor (bFGF) is also a potent neurotrophic agent increasing the outgrowth of neurites and their branching. It has been shown on fetal hippocampal neurons that under its influence the cells display larger $[Ca^{2+}]_i$ transients in response to membrane depolarization due to increased activity of L-type Ca^{2+} channels, especially at the neurite branching points, the activity of T-type remaining unchanged. The effects of increased Ca^{2+} influx on morphogenesis in this case are also mediated by changes in RNA and protein synthesis (Shitaka *et al.* 1996).

Quantitative analysis has revealed a quite sophisticated relationship between the properties of developing neuronal processes and the level of Ca^{2+} ions triggering their outgrowth. Thus, neurites formed at lower concentrations of Ca^{2+} in the presence of Mg^{2+} and NGF were found to be thinner and longer than those formed at higher concentrations of Ca^{2+} (Koike 1983; Holliday and Spitzer 1993). Thus $[Ca^{2+}]_i$ transients seem to be specially required for regulation of the rate of neurite extension (Williams and Cohan 1995). Very specific changes in calcium homeostasis occur in the growth cones. The concentration of free Ca^{2+} has been shown to influence many components of growth-cone behaviour, including the extension of filopodia and veils, the addition of new membranes to the plasmalemma, the retraction and disappearance of filopodia, and finally the collapse of the cone. Very local calcium changes in the cone have been suggested to underlie their steering by gradients of neurotransmitters and cell adhesion molecules. Depolarization caused $[Ca^{2+}]_i$ to increase at the most distal, leading tip of the growth cone. Mobile growth cones were shown to demonstrate higher $[Ca^{2+}]_i$ at their tips (Cohan *et al.* 1987). Combining a sophisticated technique for focal stimulation of growth cones with those for measuring calcium signals in single filopodia, it has been demonstrated that even single filopodia can respond to imposed stimuli independently from each other. Moreover, filopodia and their parent growth cones appear to represent functionally distinct domains of calcium regulation, possessing distinct calcium stores and sinks. Calcium stores were found to be one of the components of growth-cone calcium regulation; spatial distribution of corresponding organelles serving as morphological correlates of such localized responses—while the majority of organelles were located in the central core of the growth cone proper, peripheral organelles were detected on the base of a subset of filopodia (Davenport *et al.* 1996).

A detailed analysis of the regulation of neuronal growth-cone filopodia has been made on snail neurons. A rise in $[Ca^{2+}]_i$ induced by application of K^+-elevated solution in the filopodia caused two distinct concentration-dependent effects separable by their different time courses—within the first 10 min filopodia underwent significant elongation, while the second phase was characterized by a massive loss of filopodia. Both types of behaviour increased in a calcium-dependent fashion. In addition there were signs of a form of adaptation of filopodial behaviour to sustained $[Ca^{2+}]_i$ levels, while transient changes in $[Ca^{2+}]_i$ of as little as 30–50 nM reliably altered filopodial morphology (Rehder and Kater 1992). It should be noted that according to data on neuroblastoma cells, agents that disrupt calcium-induced calcium release did not affect calcium dynamics in the cone, indicating that local release of $[Ca^{2+}]_i$ at the tip may not be the triggering factor for the indicated processes. In contrast, L-type Ca^{2+} channels were found at higher density at the distal tip than in the proximal growth cone, suggesting the leading role of Ca^{2+} influx in the production of local transients (Amato *et al.* 1996; Zimprich and Bolsover 1995, 1996). However, observations on growth cones from DRG neurons have indicated spontaneous and transient elevations of $[Ca^{2+}]_i$ due to Ca^{2+} influx through non-voltage-gated Ca^{2+} channels as well as Ca^{2+} release and buffering by intracellular stores. Growth-cone migration was immediately and transiently inhibited during appearance of such complex $[Ca^{2+}]_i$ spikes, but eventually returned to prespike growth rates. No such spikes were observed in neuronal cell bodies or non-neuronal cells (Gomez *et al.* 1995).

The formation of neurites obviously requires the assembly of parallel arrays of microtubules that run longitudinally through neurites. Microtubules are assembled from α- and β-tubulins together with microtubule-associated proteins, and their rate of synthesis must be correlated with neurite outgrowth. It has been shown on differentiating neuroblastoma cells that α_1-tubulin mRNA level increases during neurite outgrowth, a maximal induction (1.7-fold over the initial level) occurring 24 h after neurite outgrowth onset. By contrast, when neurite outgrowth became inhibited by contact with CNS myelin, the α_1-tubulin mRNA levels show no such increase (Knoops and Octave 1997). The mechanism of such negative regulation can be only hypothetized; it may involve some silencing genes.

It should be noted that many factors may influence the time-course of neuronal differentiation and outgrowth of neurites, often leading to developmental abnormalities. Thus, overexpression of interleukin-6 (IL-6) in the central nervous system has been shown to cause extensive neuronal abnormality in mice that becomes more evident with maturation. Analysis of the effect of IL-6 treatment on rat cerebellar granule neurons in culture has shown the development of large depolarization- or transmitter-induced Ca^{2+} transients that are normally observed only in immature cells; their persistence seemed to be due to enlarged participation of calcium-induced calcium release (CICR) in the calcium response to stimulation (Holliday *et al.* 1995). A definite promoting action on neuronal differentiation is exerted by interferons. Increase in the growth of dendrites and neurites of cultured cortical and hippocampal neurons is exerted by γ-interferon (Improta *et al.* 1988; Barish *et al.* 1991). *a*2-interferon, and 2′,5′-oligoadenylate (2-5A) as an intermediate in the action of interferon, induced a more than 5-fold increase in the mean total length of neurites of differentiating neuroblastoma cells. Quite important is the fact that the effect of human *a*2-interferon was species-specific and occurred only in human (IMR-32) but not in murine (N1E-115) neuroblastoma lines; this specificity was lost at the level of oligoadenylates (Vyatchenko-Karpinskii *et al.* 1995*a*). Arachidonic acid can also stimulate neurite outgrowth, being generated by the activity of phospholipase A_2 (PLA_2). In this case it may serve as a second messenger for the activation of Ca^{2+} channels, as the induction of outgrowth could be inhibited by N- and L-channel antagonists (Williams *et al.* 1994).

An essential role in the outgrowth of neurites and their guidance is played by the local microenvironment in which this process is taking place. It is currently believed that specific guidance cues are present in the surrounding cellular environment which interact with recognition molecules on the surface of neuronal growth cones. The idea that axon guidance can be mediated by diffusible chemo-attractants was expressed by Ramon y Cajal as long ago as 1892. Over the last few years the exploration of this problem has advanced dramatically, and several chemoattractant protein molecules has been purified (see review by Keynes and Cook 1995). Among them netrin-1 and netrin-2 are best analysed as possible diffusible messengers that stimulate neurite outgrowth exerting a long-range action. At the samc timc thcy may providc bifunctional guidance, preventing axons from entering certain structures. In the extra-cellular matrix several types of macromolecule with neurite-promoting properties (laminin, tenascin, type IV collagen) were identified; laminin being the best studied and most potent. It is widely distributed in different animal species; it has been analysed in detail in the leech where it also seems to be the major neurite promoting factor (Masuda-Nakagawa *et al.* 1988).

Molecules on the surface of growing neurites which are responsible for cell adhesion (CAMs) have also been identified; among them Ca^{2+}-dependent and Ca^{2+}-independent cell adhesion glyco-protein molecules, which have been studied in detail (Takeichi 1987; Doherty *et al.* 1991; Doherty and Walsh 1991). The expression of CAMs is seen in a variety of embryonic neuronal and glial cells (N-CAMs); antibodies to these have been shown to inhibit neurite outgrowth over monolayer cultures. At the same time, substantial quantitative differences and complicated interactions were found in the effects of both molecules. In accordance with these data, neurite outgrowth responses stimulated by cell adhesion molecules were lost when a kinase-deleted, dominant negative form of fibroblast growth-factor receptors (FGFRs) were expressed in neuronal cells. In experiments of Saffell *et al.* (1997) transgenic mice were generated that expressed such dominant negative FGFRs. Cerebellar neurons isolated from these mice have lost their ability to respond to N-CAMs and other adhesion molecules. In normal mice a peptide inhibitor of phospolipase C (PLCγ) inhibited neurite outgrowth stimulated both by FGF and CAMs, indicating that activation of FGFRs is both necessary and sufficient to account for the ability of CAMs to stimulate axonal growth and that PLC is a key link in this response.

The axonal growth is connected with concomitant proliferation of related glial (astrocytic) cells. For instance, it has been shown that purified retinal ganglion cells stimulate DNA synthesis in optic nerve astrocytes in culture (Burne and Raff 1997). This effect seems to be dependent on axonal transport and not on axonal electrical activity and could be mimicked by application of the basic fibroblast growth factor (bFGF). bFGF is synthesized by developing ganglion neurons; however, it has yet to be determined if it is transported by axonal transport and released from them.

TARGET FINDING

Growing neurites have to establish future connections with different target neurons, including those with both excitatory and inhibitory functions; nevertheless, the initial suggestion that gradients of excitatory synaptic transmitters may be dominant in triggering calcium signals in growth cones and guiding their progression was found to be wrong. γ-aminobutyrate (GABA) was found to act in an excitatory manner on developing neurites of hypothalamic neurons, independently raising $[Ca^{2+}]_i$ in their growth cones. In some neurites and growth cones during early development GABA generated an even greater rise in calcium levels than did glutamate (Obrietan and Van den Pol 1996).

If a transmitter gradient is one guidance cue for growing nerve processes, then growth cones should exhibit some kind of chemotaxic behaviour *in vivo* or in cell culture: turning in the direction of a defined gradient. In fact it has been shown on cell cultures of isolated embryonic spinal neurons of *Xenopus* that their growth cones demonstrate such turning responses in a defined gradient of acetylcholine (ACh). The response depends on activation of neuronal nicotinic ACh receptors and requires the presence of extracellular Ca^{2+}. The growth cones showed a small but significant elevation of $[Ca^{2+}]_i$ within minutes of the onset of ACh application and before the beginning of turning. Higher elevations of $[Ca^{2+}]_i$ induced growth inhibition or neurite retraction. The effect seems to be mediated by Ca^{2+}-calmodulin-dependent protein kinase II, as it could be completely inhibited by specific CaM kinase II inhibitor KN62 (Zheng *et al.* 1994). Dynamic distal ends of microtubules in the growth cones seem to play a key role in the actin filament-mediated strewing of growth-cone microtubules producing growth-cone turning (Challacombe *et al.* 1997).

Another factor important for axon guidance has been shown to be the receptor tyrosine kinases (RTKs), specially their so-called Eph subfamily (cf. review by Brambilla and Klein 1995). These receptors were found to be highly over-expressed in an erythropoietin-producing hepatocellular carcinoma cell line and therefore designated as Eph. Most of these receptors are predominantly expressed in the developing nervous system. Several ligands were identified which bind to the extracellular portion of the receptors and induce their autophosphorylation. In experiments on cortical neuron–astrocyte co-cultures it has been shown that signals transduced by the Eph receptors do not induce cell differentiation—they only steer growing axons away from incorrect targets rather than attracting them to correct ones. In mutant mice lacking brain-derived neurotrophic factor (BDNF), one of the ligands for tyrosin kinase receptor B, the developing taste buds lacked up to 98 per cent of innervation by taste neurons, while absence of other neurotrophins (NT3, NT4) did not exert such an effect (Zhang *et al.* 1997). There are indications that activation of tyrosine-kinase in some cases can induce even an opposite effect on cell differentiation; thus in PC12 pheochromocytoma cells inhibition of protein RTK *increased* the rate of neurite elongation when it had been primed with NGF (Miller *et al.* 1993). Recent data indicate that the influence of BDNF and subsequent activation of RTK B may be quite specific in nature. It has been shown on hippocampal slices from P12–P18 old rats that it did not exert any appreciable effect on evoked excitatory postsynaptic responses, but markedly reduced both the evoked and spontaneous inhibitory ($GABA_A$-mediated) responses (Tanaka *et al.* 1997). It has been suggested by the authors that such disinhibition would enhance synaptic activity important for developmental changes.

Eph receptors expressed on astrocytes are also not a favourable substrate, and the axons prefer to grow on top of each other rather than on astrocytes, thus producing bundles of nerve fibres. However, the signal transduction mechanism downstream of the Eph receptors still has to be elucidated.

The most important question is also the nature of events which happen when the growing axon first contacts its target cell. This question has been addressed both on nerve-muscle and interneuronal contacts. A consistent finding was an increase of Ca^{2+} influx in the presynaptic structure and elevation of presynaptic $[Ca^{2+}]_i$ level (Funte and Haydon 1993; Dai and Peng 1993). The elevation occurred very rapidly (within 30 min) and could be blocked by addition of cAMP-dependent protein kinase inhibitor H-7. In contrast, addition of dbcAMP to the culture reversibly enhanced calcium accumulation. It could also be suppressed by lifting the nerve terminal away from the myoball, by addition of Ca^{2+}-free extracellular solution, and by addition of polyanionic compounds that interfere with cell-surface receptors. Presynaptic $[Ca^{2+}]_i$ elevation in many connections was positive for induction of neurotransmission while its suppression was accompanied by a reduction of transmitter release. Morphological changes also occur at this time—neurite extension stops, and structures typical of the presynaptic terminals develop. All these findings indicate that the target substrate released some signals which retrogradely regulate calcium homeostasis in presynaptic nerve terminals, an important link there being the activation of cAMP-dependent protein kinase. The molecules mediating the contact-induced $[Ca^{2+}]_i$ elevation are not known. Several studies have shown that there is a strong adhesive interaction between both cells, in which the already mentioned cell adhesion molecules may play a role; extracellular matrix proteins (laminin and others) may also be important. A recent finding from dissociated cochlear neurons from rat embryos has shown an important role in this respect of one member of the NGF family—neurotrophin-3—which might be released from the differentiating sensory epithelium of the cochlea. Neurons isolated at embryonic days 7–11 and maintained for 2 d in culture with neurotrophin-3 showed a substantial increase in Ca^{2+} current density, particularly in its transient component (Jimenez *et al.* 1997).

It should be taken into account that the progressing growth cone, even before its contact with the target cell, can already release transmitters which may also participate in the complex machinery of the formation of synaptic junctions. This has been shown on dorsal root ganglion neurons growing in culture containing acutely dissociated hippocampal neurons with glutamate receptors. Inward currents were recorded in the latter if they were positioned on the growth cones while Ca^{2+} ion concentration increased in the latter in response to DRG neuron stimulation. Thus the growth cones are already endowed with much of the machinery for neurotransmitter release before making a corresponding structure (Soeda *et al.* 1997).

The inhibition of neuronal differentiation induced by establishment of a contact with its target is also a calcium-dependent process. Extracellular Ca^{2+} is necessary for this process, which seems to be mediated by the synthesis of some inhibitory factor. This factor does not appear to be toxic to cultured cells and thus does not decrease the number of neurons through death; it appears only to suppress or delay neuronal differentiation (Holliday and Spitzer 1993).

Figure 1.5 presents in schematic form the main cellular mechanisms which determine the onset of cell differentiation, the outgrowth of neurites, and the direction of their elongation.

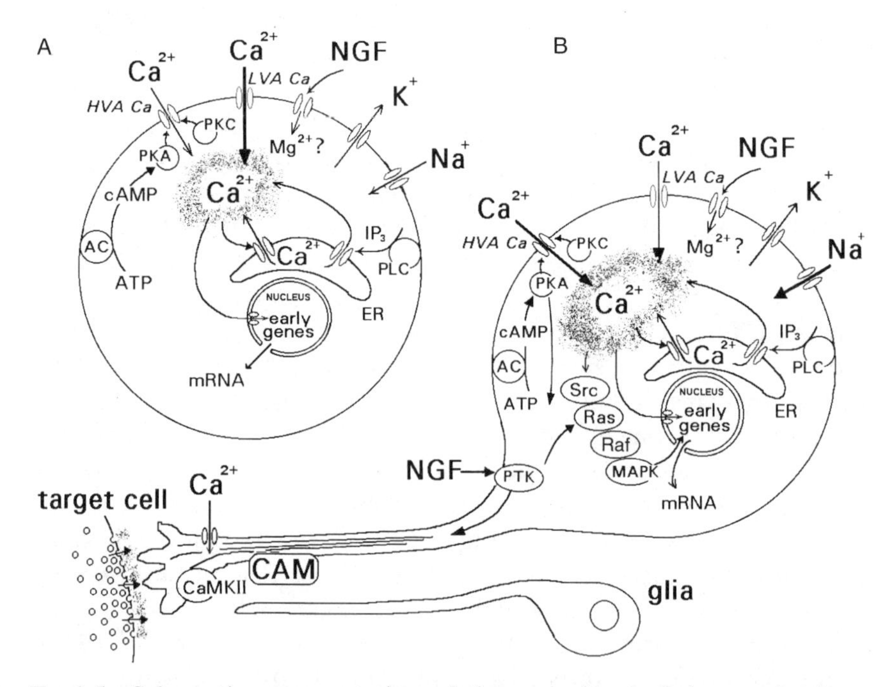

FIG 1.5 Schematic representation of the main intracellular mechanisms responsible for the beginning of cell differentiation (A) and outgrowth of neurites (B). *LVA Ca* and *HVA Ca*–low- and high-voltage-activated Ca^{2+} channels, NGF–nerve-growth factors, PKA and PKC–corresponding protein kinases, AC–adenylate cyclase, PLC–phospholipase C, Src–non-receptor tyrosine kinase, Ras–GTP-binding proteins, Raf-cytoplasmic serine threonin kinase, MAPK–mitogen-activated protein kinase, CaM kinase II–calcium-calmodulin-dependent kinase, RTK–receptor tyrosine kinase, CAM–cell adhesion molecules.

EFFECTS OF AXOTOMY

Complicated changes in neuronal properties can occur also in the opposite situation—when the intercellular contact is destroyed (for instance, by axotomy). Detailed analysis of this question is outside the scope of this monograph; in general it should be mentioned that according to several investigations axotomy in mature neurons provokes marked changes in their morphological, biochemical, and electrophysiolgical properties due to lack of retrograde trophic influences from the target cells. In neurons innervating peripheral targets some of these changes lead to axon degeneration, and if the cell bodies do not successfully reinnervate a target, death is usually the final outcome. Again one of the prominent alterations in the axotomized neurons is a change in Ca^{2+} homeostasis. It has been shown that regeneration of neurites and formation of growth cones in *Helisoma* neurons was *delayed* by elevated $[Ca^{2+}]_i$ (Rehder *et al.* 1992). According to recent measurements on rat axotomized sympathetic ganglion cells, 7–10 d after section no substantial differences occur in their resting $[Ca^{2+}]_i$ level. However, the rise in $[Ca^{2+}]_i$ evoked by orthodromic or antidromic stimulation and the recovery after stimulation were considerably slowed down. This slowing of calcium dynamics could be due to changes in buffering capacity of the axotomized cells as well as to changes in Ca^{2+} influx. Changes in membrane properties were also observed in such cells: often the action potentials were followed by after-depolarizations instead of the after-hyperpolarizations that are always present in healthy cells. A conclusion can be made that moderate increases in intracellular calcium levels may play a role in the regenerative responses and in survival after trophic factor deprivation, while higher levels may be involved in neuronal death which would follow if the cell does not recover its normal retrograde supply of trophic factors (Sanchez-Vives and Gallego 1993; Sanchez-Vives *et al.* 1994). Basic fibroblast growth factor can be helpful in increasing cell survival and supporting axonal re-elongation if applied after axotomy; this has been shown in *in vitro* experiments and even has been suggested as a new therapeutic concept for management of axonal injury in patients (Himmelseher *et al.* 1997). In contrast, re-establishment of synaptic connections in the hypothalamic CA3 region after a lesion of mossy fibres can be hindered by epileptic activity (elicited by picrotoxin); however this inhibitory effect could be completely abolished by tetrodotoxin or the L-type Ca^{2+} channel-blocker nicardipine, indicating that in this case excessive influx of Ca^{2+} via L-type channels during epileptic bursts can also mediate the disturbance of appropriate synapse formation by mossy fibres (Ikegava *et al.* 1997).

Deafferented neurons also may undergo apoptosis, and it has been shown recently *in vivo* on bird motor-cortical neurons that neurotrophins can prevent such death (Johnson *et al.* 1997). Obviously, in this case non-retrograde signalling by neurotrophins may promote neuron survival; however, the mechanisms of this signalling and of its action on the deafferented neurons have to be determined.

If the neuron survives, the problem of re-establishment of connections with target cells during reinnervation is definitely much more complicated than embryonic development of the system. The growth cones again have to find their way, using turning, collapse, and retraction in response to different extracellular matrix molecules. The failure of neurons to regenerate following injury is due in part to the interaction of the growth cone with molecules present on the surface of oligodendrocytes as myelin-forming cells and is seen in the form of collapse and retraction of the neuronal growth cones after contact with them. The inhibitory effect of myelin might be mediated by several intermediates, like the neurite growth inhibitor NI-35, which inhibits regeneration of lesioned neuronal fibres *in vivo* and growth of neurites *in v*itro (Bandtlow *et al.* 1993). Certain specificity has been observed in this process: for instance, growth cones of neonatal rat brain stem neurons in culture collapsed following contact with central myelin, but continued to elongate on contact with peripheral myelin. The mechanism of this action again seems to be of the same general nature: central myelin elicited a substantial (about 3-fold) increase in $[Ca^{2+}]_i$ in these growth cones and their collapse, while peripheral myelin did not. The increase required trans-membrane Ca^{2+} influx, since it could be blocked by extracellular EGTA (ethylenebis(oxyethylenenitrilo)tetraacetic acid) and by application of ω-conotoxin GVIA, a specific blocker of N-type Ca^{2+} channels (Moorman and Hume 1993). A similar role can be played also by gradients of chemical transmitters: it has been shown on isolated ciliary neurons in culture that retraction of their growing processes can be induced by activation, by acetylcholine, of extrasynaptic nicotinic chemoreceptors present on their surface. The retraction in this case also requires extracellular Ca^{2+}. Obviously the resulting membrane depolarization again activates Ca^{2+} channels which permit a sufficient amount of Ca^{2+} ions to enter the neurite to prevent further outgrowth and induce retraction (Pugh and Berg 1994). Substantial changes might occur also in the extracellular surroundings of the regenerating axons in form of accumulation of laminin and other matrix molecules, attraction of microglial cells, etc. (Masuda-Nakagawa *et al.* 1990)

Despite all the problems that face the regenerating axon, the process of re-establishing synaptic connection in a neuronal network can proceed quite rapidly. Special observations on lesion-induced neurite sprouting and synapse formation in hippocampal organotypic culture have shown that formation of new functional synaptic contacts and complete recovery of transmission can take place within 3–6 d. Interestingly, functional recovery in cultures of older cells (3 weeks old) was found to be significantly slower than that in one-week-old tissue (Stoppini *et al.* 1993).

OUTGROWTH OF DENDRITES

Much less is known about mechanisms responsible for the regulation of the outgrowth and maturation of the dendritic tree of nerve cells. Recently it became possible to use time-lapse fluorescent microscopy to visualize directly the formation and dynamics of dendritic branches and spines in developing hippocampal tissue slices (Dailey and Smith 1996). It has been shown that within 2 weeks the pyramidal neurons in cultured slices from early postnatal rat (2nd–7th postnatal days) developed a complex dendritic arbor bearing numerous dendritic spines. At the beginning the dendritic shaft carried many fine filopodial protrusions which extended rapidly (maximum rate about 2.5 $\mu m\ min^{-1}$) and retracted. However, some transformed themselves into growth-cone-like structures and formed dendrite branches. As the dendritic arbors matured, the population of fleeting lateral filopodia replaced themselves by spine-like structures having a low rate of turnover. This developmental period involved a transitional stage in which the dendrites were dominated by persistent (up to 22 h) but dynamic spiny protrusions ('protospines') that showed substantial changes in length and shape on a time scale of minutes. Obviously, these changes, in parallel with the above described changes in the axonal terminals may actively contribute to the formation and plasticity of synaptic connections during the development of neuronal networks. The labile dendritic protrusions might actually be involved in establishing axo-dendritic synaptic contacts. Of course, it would be quite important in the future to learn how the motility of developing dendrites is generated and regulated and what kind of surface molecules are responsible for the recognition of the appropriate axonal partners and the initiation of corresponding synaptogenesis. In experiments on developing hippocampal neurons *in vitro* it has been shown that glutamate release is crucial for the onset of dendritic morphology, most prominently reflected in the length of the terminal dendritic segments. Chronic addition of ionotropic glutamate receptor antagonists from day 2 in culture arrested dendritic development at the prefunctional level (Nuijtinck *et al.* 1997).

PROGRAMMED DEATH

The programmed death of neurons which did not establish connections with target cells during development is also important in the formation of neuronal networks; it seems that all factors which promote survival are in fact not stimulating life but suppressing the death programme. Such promotion is a complicated event which depends both on the action of growth factors and on intracellular Ca^{2+}. It has been shown by many authors that neuronal survival at early developmental stages can be induced by elevation of extracellular level of K^+ ions and membrane depolarization which promote influx of Ca^{2+} and elevation of $[Ca^{2+}]_i$ by 2–3 times; the same effect could be induced by thapsigargin which blocks the sequestration of Ca^{2+} by intracellular stores (Johnson and Deckwerth 1993; Franklin *et al.* 1995; Lampe *et al.* 1995). Developmental increase in the resting intracellular level of Ca^{2+} may form a mechanism which decreases the dependence of cell on trophic factors with maturation. This machinery has been effectively studied on embryonic neurons developing in culture (cf. review by Franklin and Johnson 1994). At very low $[Ca^{2+}]_i$ most neurons cannot survive in culture even in the presence of NGF. At resting level (60–100 nM) the survival becomes acutely dependent on NGF, and modest elevations of $[Ca^{2+}]_i$ (50–70 nM above the resting level) promote survival in the absence of NGF. However, the promoting concentration window ('life or death set-point') appears to be very narrow, and higher levels of $[Ca^{2+}]_i$ as well as prolonged exposure to high potassium concentrations may exert a toxic effect (Kawasaki *et al.* 1988). Similar data have recently been obtained from cultured spiral ganglion neurons from neonatal rats. $[Ca^{2+}]_i$ elevated to 250–350 nM enabled neuronal survival independent of exogenous neurotrophic factors, while higher $[Ca^{2+}]_i$ was associated with cell death (Hegarty *et al.* 1997). An interesting point is the absence of a connection between the effects of elevated $[Ca^{2+}]_i$ on neuronal survival and the continuation of differentiation. While chronic depolarization promoted survival of neurons even in the absence of NGF, the cells supported in this manner showed little growth as measured by neurite extension and mean somatic diameter (Franklin *et al.* 1995). This finding corresponds to the already mentioned narrow window of intracellular Ca^{2+} in which stimulation of neurite outgrowth takes place.

The action of neurotrophins may be also of opposite character. It has been shown recently that NGF and other neurotrophins can bind to receptors with different affinity; binding to the low affinity ones (marked as $p75^{NTR}$) may lead in some cases to apoptotic events in a very cell-type-specific manner (cf. review by Carter and Lewin 1997) The intrinsic mechanisms of this complicated interaction are still not settled. The participation of PKC and PKA (protein kinase A) as well as the involvement of calmodulin has been suggested, as elevation of the intracellular level of cAMP is also a factor which promotes survival (Michel and Agid 1996). In favour of these mechanisms are the observations that pituitary adenylate cyclase-activating polypeptide (PACAP-38), a member of the vasoactive intestinal peptide (VIP) family, protects cerebellar granule neurons from apoptosis in culture by cAMP-dependent activation of the mitogen-activated protein kinase pathway, the important role of which in neuronal development has been already mentioned (Villalba *et al.* 1977). On the other hand, the elevated cytoplasmic $[Ca^{2+}]_i$ necessary for the development of K^+-dependent survival of superior cervical ganglion cells *in vitro* has been shown to depend on up-regulation of the expression of L-type Ca^{2+} channels under the influence of NGF (Tanaka and Koike 1995). It has to be kept in mind that because of opposite effect of excessive $[Ca^{2+}]_i$ elevation, under certain conditions Ca^{2+}-channel blockers may be beneficial for survival (cf. Landfield 1996).

Other intracellular pathways independent on high-K^+-induced elevation of $[Ca^{2+}]_i$ may also mediate neuronal survival. It has been shown recently that cultured cerebellar granule neurons can survive even in a low-K^+ medium if subjected to the insulin-like growth factor (IGF-1) which activates phosphoinositide 3-kinase (PI 3-

kinase). It has been suggested that IGF-1-mediated activation of PI 3-kinase leads to a suppression of 'killer gene' expression (D'Mello *et al.* 1997).

Ca^{2+} overload may trigger apoptosis of the sacrificed cells by several enzymatic mechanisms. These include endonuclease-mediated cleavage of DNA, topoisomerase-mediated DNA fragmentation, and subsequent activation of Ca^{2+}-activated proteases which affect cytoskeletal elements and membrane integral proteins, etc.

CONCLUSIONS

The formation of neuronal networks is an extremely complicated process which includes several interconnected steps triggered by external and intracellular signals. Elevation of intracellular Ca^{2+} is the most important even at the initial step—migration of neuronal precursors to the site of their destination and induction of the outgrowth of neurites. LVA Ca^{2+} channels here play a prominent role as they can trigger intracellular Ca^{2+} waves and spikes at membrane potentials close to the resting level. Ca^{2+} release from stores may substantially amplify these signals. This triggering mechanism is extremely sensitive and functions in a narrow window of $[Ca^{2+}]_i$; higher levels induce retraction of processes and collapse of growth cones, in which the changes of Ca^{2+} homeostasis are especially sophisticated. Phosphorylation–dephosphorylation of cyto-skeletal proteins are the immediate mechanisms of the action of Ca^{2+}, changes in gene expression being responsible for more long-lasting effects. Nerve-growth factors are the most important external triggers, also involving changes in intracellular Ca^{2+}; cell-adhesion molecules and neurotransmitter gradients help in guiding the growing axons. After establishing synaptic contacts, specific elevations of $[Ca^{2+}]_i$ in the presynaptic terminals induced by some retrograde messengers are responsible for their maturation and induction of synaptic transmission. Similar events may occur during reinnervation after axotomy, provided that the parent neuron survived the retrograde degenerative processes.

2

Developmental plasticity of neuronal elements

GENERAL FEATURES

The formation of neuronal networks is connected with simultaneous developmental changes in the functional properties of neuronal elements which have to match the new tasks they have to fulfil. These changes have been studied in numerous investigations carried out both on cells *in situ* and on persistent cell cultures as well as on differentiating malignant cell lines. Voltage- and ligand-operated ion channels, as well as intracellular messenger systems, definitely undergo changes during neuronal ontogenesis; they can be both of a quantitative nature, expressed in modifications of their expression in different types of cell as well as in different parts of the same cell, and of a qualitative nature. A very general estimate of these changes can made by autoradiographic analysis of the animal brain during post-natal ontogenesis using different channel markers, for instance radioactively-labelled TTX, apamin, and verapamil as indicators of the presence of sodium, Ca^{2+}-dependent potassium, and L-type calcium channels, respectively. No TTX binding has been detected at birth, and its appearance correlated with synaptogenesis. Apamin receptors were present at birth, and their density increased up to 20 d. Verapamil receptors developed later, probably following the development of dendrites, and regularly increased in density until adulthood (cf. Mourre *et al.* 1987). However, the developmental changes can be followed much more precisely by using direct recordings of the corresponding currents from different neuronal structures.

DIFFERENT TYPES OF CALCIUM CHANNEL

The most extensively analysed are the developmental changes in the spectrum and density of voltage-operated Ca^{2+} channels (VOCCs).

A constant feature here is the change in representation of the two main categories of these channels—low- and high-voltage-activated (HVA and LVA); the first are highly expressed during early ontogenesis and disappear with maturation, the second become dominant in adult cells. Very convenient objects for revealing these changes are not neuronal cells but skeletal and cardiac muscle fibres. The LVA Ca^{2+} channels are dominant in embryonic chick cardiomyocytes (Kawano and DeHaan 1991) and skeletal muscle fibres (Adams and Beam 1989; Kano *et al.* 1991), but they disappeared when the growth rate of fibres approached zero (Xu and Best 1992). More precisely these changes during the early postnatal period have been followed in rat ventricular cardiomyocytes: on the 2nd day both LVA and HVA Ca^{2+} currents could be evoked in their membrane, while on the 7th day only HVA (L-type) currents could be evoked (Gomez *et al.* 1994). The simplest explanation of the functional meaning of the early appearance of low-voltage-activated Ca^{2+} currents in ontogenesis is the triggering of membrane depolarization waves which in turn elicit activation of HVA Ca^{2+} channels and generation of intracellular Ca^{2+} transients necessary for stimulating morphogenesis (Spitzer *et al.* 1992). Myocytes also demonstrate other developmental changes in intracellular mechanisms which are connected to the functioning of 'adult' Ca^{2+} channels: in early stages of development the L-type Ca^{2+} channels are insensitive to β-adrenergic modulation and cAMP, probably because of absence or low expression of the corresponding protein kinase and also some other elements in the signalling cascade (An *et al.* 1996). With the accomplishment of differentiation this cascade becomes active; however, at its opposite end modifications occur in the functional properties of the adenylate cyclase complex manifested by a decrease in its capacity to be stimulated by post-receptor mechanisms including GTP-binding proteins (Morris and Bilezikian 1986) and probable decrease in its tonic inhibition by G_i-proteins (Osaka and Joyner 1992).

In neuronal cells the coincidence of the predominant expression of LVA channels with cell maturation was first demonstrated on rat DRG neurons (Fedulova *et al.* 1985, 1986; Kostyuk *et al.* 1986). Well expressed in cells from neonatal animals, these channels start to decline rapidly in density with maturation. At the age of 3 months, when the differentiation of sensory neurons is accomplished, 80 per cent of isolated cells did not have any LVA-channel activity, Ca^{2+} conductance being represented only by HVA channels. In contrast,

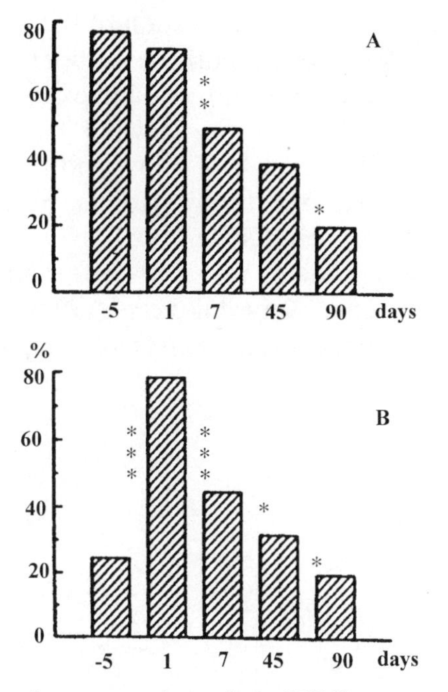

FIG 2.1 Changes in the proportion of rat DRG neurons revealing LVA Ca^{2+} (A) and slow TTX-insensitive Na^{+} (B) currents. Abscissa–days before and after birth; ordinate–percentage of cells. Asterisks indicate significance levels (from Fedulova *et al.* 1994).

when followed during prenatal development, LVA channels were expressed in about 80 per cent of tested cells (Fedulova *et al.* 1994). The statistical data about described developmental changes in the expression of LVA Ca^{2+} channels in rat primary sensory neurons are illustrated in Fig. 2.1.

In cultured embryonic sensory neurons from *Xenopus* LVA Ca^{2+} channels were expressed only during the first 20–40 h of culture (Barish 1991). *In vivo* observations on differentiating spinal cord neurons from embryos of the same animal also showed a temporal increase in density of LVA (T-type) Ca^{2+} currents before maturation (Desarmenien *et al.* 1993).

Temporal appearance of LVA Ca^{2+} channels in the early postnatal period has been demonstrated in other neuronal structures. Retinal ganglion neurons investigated between the 14th embryonic (E14) and 25th postnatal (P25) days did not reveal Ca^{2+} currents before E17; later on only LVA currents became expressed, and they were eliminated with the onset of HVA currents which steadily increased in density with development, maturation of the electrical properties of the cells not being achieved until the rat opened its eyes (Schmid and Guenther 1996). Similar progression in expression of HVA Ca^{2+} currents was observed in *in situ* developing cerebellar granule neurons, which at P14 consisted of a fast and slow component and, after P19, of a slow component only (Rossi *et al.* 1994). In rat visual cortical neurons LVA currents were well expressed at day P2, but disappeared at P12, being replaced by rapidly increasing in amplitude HVA currents (Tarasenko *et al.* 1998).

Figure 2.2 illustrates these extremely rapid developmental

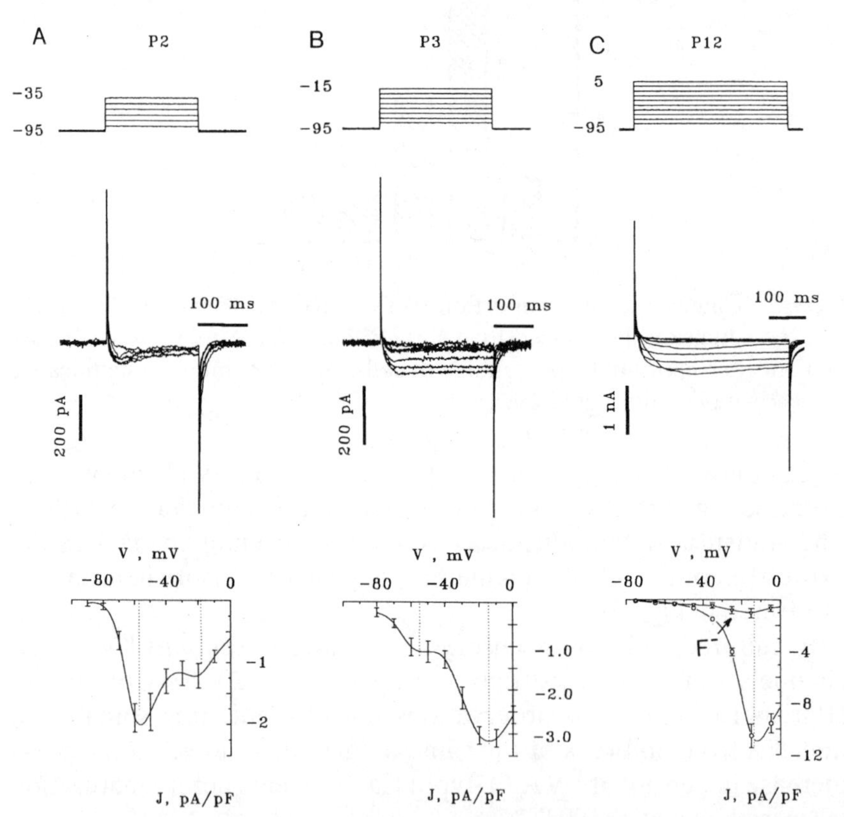

FIG 2.2 Whole-cell Ca^{2+} currents in neurons from rat visual cortex (layer V–VI) recorded at postnatal days P2 (A), P3 (B) and P12 (C). In each panel the voltage protocols are shown at the top, the current traces in the middle and I–V relationships below. Note the typical hump in the I–V curves from P2 and P3 neurons, separating the maxima of LVA and HVA Ca^{2+} currents, and its absence at P12. The HVA Ca^{2+} currents in C could be almost completely blocked by intracellular injection of fluoride (Tarasenko *et al.* 1998).

changes in the expression of both types of Ca^{2+} channel in rat visual cortex neurons. It has to be mentioned that LVA Ca^{2+} currents here could be found only in neurons of the deep (V–VI) and superficial (I) layers; in the middle layer (II–III) neurons only HVA Ca^{2+} currents could be recorded, even at days P2–P3.

In rat and guinea-pig hippocampal pyramidal neurons LVA currents were found only in the immature state; they could not be detected in cells isolated from adult animals (O'Dell and Alger 1991; Thompson and Wong 1991). A similar difference was found for neurons obtained from embryonic or adult neostriatum (Bargas *et al.* 1991).

The temporary appearance of LVA Ca^{2+} channels at early developmental stages in all the above mentioned structures indicates their significance in morphogenesis. As has been already mentioned in the previous chapter, their ability to be activated close to the resting potential level makes them especially suitable for generation of intracellular Ca^{2+} transients and Ca^{2+} waves important for triggering differentiation, formation of synaptic contacts, etc. Substantial differences between the expression times of these channels in different neurons reflect differences in the time course of their maturation; one may speculate that the development of the projections of primary sensory neurons (and also thalamic neurons) is a much more time-consuming process and demands more long-lasting triggering action of the intracellular Ca^{2+} transients provided by the activity of LVA Ca^{2+} channels.

Specific changes in the expression of these main types of Ca^{2+} channel occur during the period of programmed cell death and elimination of excessive synapses: the density of HVA channels significantly increases at this time, while that of LVA channels continues to decline (Mynlieff and Beam 1992). Interestingly, very similar changes might also occur if developing neurons are chronically exposed to alcohol: it has been shown on cultured cerebellar Purkinje neurons that such treatment for 8–10 d also significantly increased the amplitude of HVA Ca^{2+} currents, especially their sustained components, while reducing the LVA currents (Gruol and Parsons 1994).

The same sequence of developmental events can be demonstrated on neurons growing in culture and on malignant cell lines subjected to differentiation. Thus chick DRG precursor cells can differentiate in culture into morphologically and functionally mature neurons. Non-differentiated proliferating cells do not reveal any substantial Ca^{2+} conductance (Kostyuk *et al.* 1978). During the first 10 h in culture they demonstrate only LVA Ca^{2+} currents which are well expressed both in soma and in growth cones; later on HVA currents start to appear. It is known for certain that in this case only the activity of LVA Ca^{2+} channels is necessary for triggering and regulation of the activity of growth cones, the early expression of HVA channels being unnecessary for this process (Veselovsky and Fomina 1986; Gottmann *et al.* 1991). DRG neuron precursors taken from E11–E13 mice also differentiate in culture. In this case activity of both LVA and HVA Ca^{2+} channels could be detected at early stages; however, the density of the former decreased later while that of the second increased dramatically (Bickmayer *et al.* 1993). In molluscan neurons the action of such differentiation-stimulating factors as NGF even on adult neurons acutely enhanced the HVA Ca^{2+} currents (Wilderling *et al.* 1995). Differentiating cells from malignant cell lines activated by NGF or similar factors demonstrate similar changes—large increases in the density of HVA currents, which include components with different pharmacological sensitivity, and disappearance of LVA currents (Lewis *et al.* 1993).

However, the expression of LVA Ca^{2+} channels during early ontogenesis is not a general rule; in some neuronal structures they remain well expressed during the whole life cycle. This developmental behaviour is found to be connected with the presence of several subtypes of LVA channels differing in functional properties and pharmacological sensitivity. The first description of a special type of LVA channel was made by Akaike *et al.* (1989) on rat hypothalamic neurons, which revealed LVA Ca^{2+} currents highly sensitive to dihydropyridines (nifedipine) and Cd^{2+} ions—a property particularly characteristic of HVA L-type Ca^{2+} channels. LVA channels with similar pharmacological sensitivity were described also in cell bodies of isolated rat cerebellar Purkinje neurons (Kaneda *et al.* 1990). We continued this analysis on neurons of the associative (latero–dorsal) thalamic nuclei and have shown that here the LVA Ca^{2+} currents can be clearly separated into two components which are differently expressed during postnatal ontogenesis. In neurons from animals at stage P12 the population of LVA Ca^{2+} channels was found to be homogeneous; the corresponding currents could be elicited by depolarizing voltage steps from holding potentials more negative than –70 mV, showed fast inactivation with a time constant of about 30 ms, and were highly sensitive to nimodipine (K_d = 2.6 μM) and Cd^{2+} (K_d about 1 μM). However, even at stages P14–P17 the population of LVA channels became heterogeneous, and a fraction of nimodipine-insensitive channels appeared with slower kinetics. The mean inactivation time-constant of the corresponding current reached 54 and 68 ms for P14 and P17 neurons, respectively. In contrast with the fast component, it could be effectively blocked by Ni^{2+} (at concentrations of 25 μM). The appearance of this component obviously coincided with dendritic expansion of the thalamic neurons, as could be judged from progressive increase of their membrane capacitance. This stage of postnatal development also corresponds to the appearance of the rhythmic thalamo–cortical activity; therefore it can be suggested that the slow LVA Ca^{2+} currents generated in the dendritic arborizations play an important role in triggering these activities in the developed brain (Tarasenko *et al.* 1997). On the other hand, dihydropyridine-sensitive channels active at the resting membrane potential level contribute to maintenance of the resting intracellular Ca^{2+} concentration, as has been demonstrated on hippocampal CA1 pyramidal neurons; these channels appeared to be present throughout the neuron and located most densely in the proximal apical dendrites (Magee *et al.* 1996).

Figure 2.3 illustrates these specific features of developmental expression of Ca^{2+} channels in neurons of the rat latero–dorsal thalamic nucleus. At the P12 stage the LVA part of the I–V relationship showed a single peak, while already at P14 two peaks became obvious with maxima at about –65 and –55 mV (Tarasenko *et al.* 1997). The two LVA Ca^{2+} current components in these neurons could be recorded separately using their different sensitivity to La^{3+} and Ni^{2+}, as is illustrated in Fig. 2.4; the La^{3+}- (and nifedipine-) sensitive component ($I_{T,f}$) reveals fast voltage-dependent inactivation, while the Ni^{2+}-sensitive component ($I_{T,s}$) is inactivated more slowly. Statistical data about the developmental expression of both types of LVA Ca^{2+} current are presented in Fig. 2.5.

LVA Ca^{2+} channels were observed also in neurons isolated from other thalamic nuclei of the adult animals: nucleus reticularis (Huguenard and Prince 1992; Tsakiridou *et al.* 1995*a*), ventrobasal complex (Coulter *et al.* 1989), as well as in cerebellar Purkinje neurons (Kaneda *et al.* 1990), and even in a population of middle-sized primary sensory neurons in the dorsal-root ganglia (Shmigol *et al.* 1995*a*). In the case of cells from the DRG neuron–neuroblastoma line LVA Ca^{2+} currents were recorded with unusually slow inactivation kinetics (Kobrinsky *et al.* 1994). However, the results obtained from enzymatically treated isolated neurons may be less

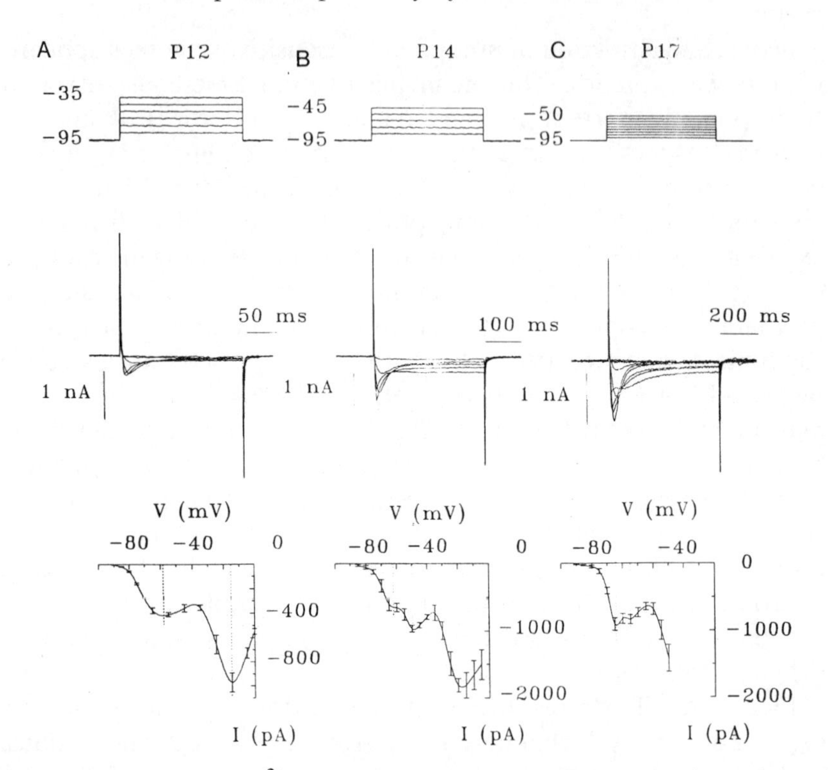

FIG 2.3 Whole-cell Ca^{2+} currents in neurons from rat dorso–lateral thalamic nucleus recorded at postnatal days P12 (A), P14 (B) and P17 (C). The figure is constructed similarly to Fig. 2.2. Note the appearance of two LVA current peaks at P14 with maxima at about –65 and –55 mV and well preserved LVA current at P17 (from Tarasenko *et al.* 1997).

representative than neurons *in situ*, when they retain their dendrites. A special analysis of this problem has been made recently on reticular thalamic neurons, using a comparison of data obtained from isolated dendrite-free cells and cells in slices with subsequent computational analysis of the effects of currents originating in distal dendrites (Destexhe *et al.* 1996). It has been shown that LVA Ca^{2+} channels on distal dendrites make a substantial contribution to the corresponding total Ca^{2+} current. In hippocampal neurons from brain slices of adult rats LVA Ca^{2+} currents were generated exclusively in terminal dendrites—superficial cuts of the tissue, leaving only the deep layers of the grey matter, completely abolished them (Karst *et al.* 1993). Dopaminergic neurons from substantia nigra *in situ* also demonstrated exceptionally high-amplitude LVA Ca^{2+} currents absent in isolated neurons (Kang and Kitai 1993)

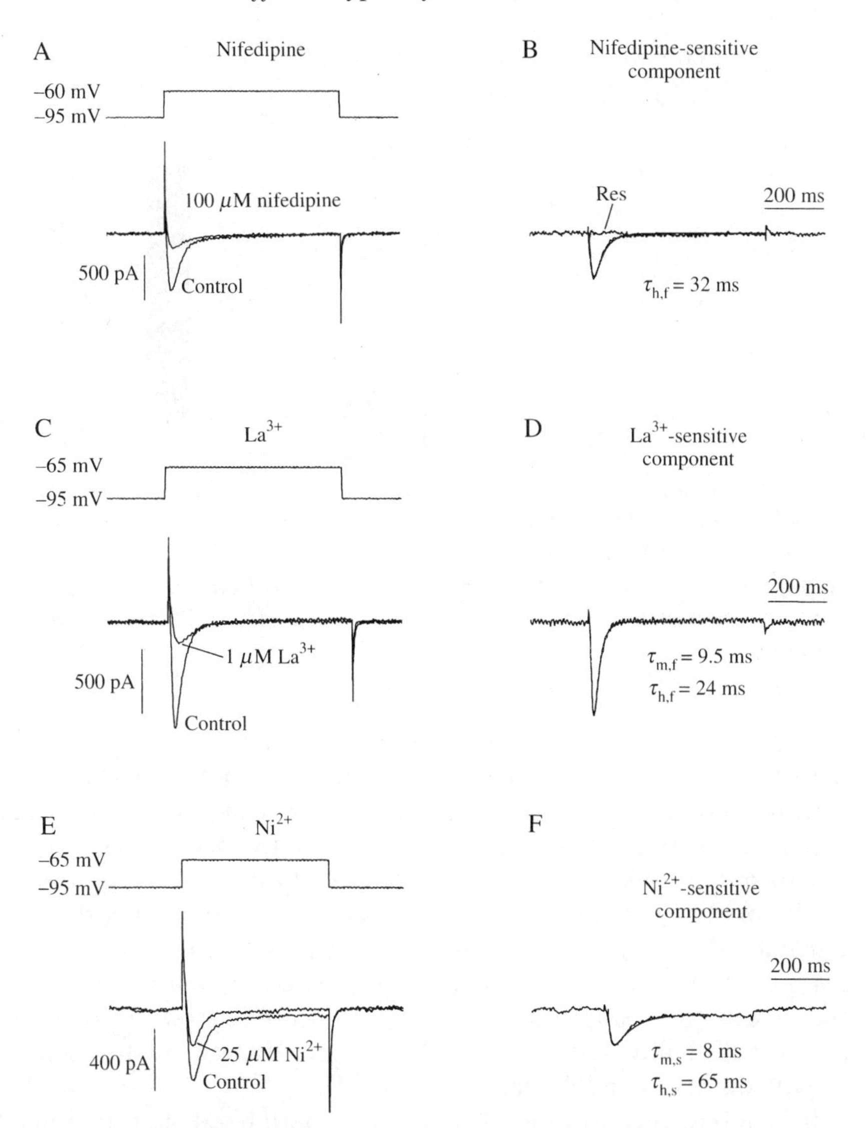

FIG 2.4 Pharmacological properties of different components of the LVA Ca^{2+} currents in LD thalamic neurons at stage P17. (A–B): LVA currents recorded before (control) and in the presence of 100 μM nifedipine; nifedipine-sensitive ('fast') component obtained by subtraction of the current recorded after addition of the drug from the control current. (C–D): similar component isolated by application of 1 μM La^{2+}. (E–F): Ni^{2+}-sensitive ('slow') component obtained in the same way by addition of 25 μM Ni^{2+}. The values of the activation (τ_m) and inactivation (τ_h) time-constants are indicated near the records. Voltage protocols are shown at the top (modified from Tarasenko *et al.* 1997).

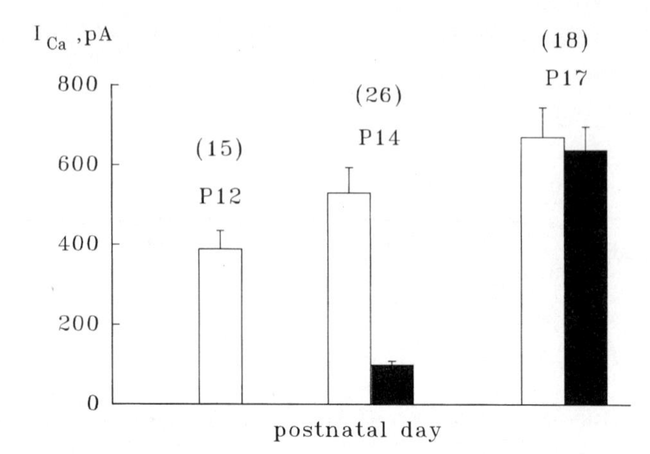

FIG 2.5 Statistical data showing developmental changes in the expression of the two components of LVA Ca^{2+} currents in neurons of the rat LD thalamic nucleus. Open columns represent $I_{T,f}$ and filled ones $I_{T,s}$. The mean amplitudes ± S.E. are plotted as a function of postnatal age. Figures in parentheses indicate the number of cells tested (from Tarasenko *et al.* 1997).

The functional role of permanently expressed LVA Ca^{2+} channels in central nervous system neurons is connected with their ability to activate low-threshold spikes subsequent to transient membrane hyperpolarization removing their steady-state inactivation. Such low-threshold spikes may then lead to burst firing and promotion of oscillatory behaviour in the neuronal thalamo–cortical networks (cf. Huguenard 1996). Substantial theoretical analysis produced a mathematical model which describes the frequency characteristics of such oscillatory behaviour and the presence of certain resonance patterns probably important for the organization of low-frequency activity during sleep (Hutcheon *et al.* 1994).

It is interesting to note that in some peripheral non-neuronal tissues LVA Ca^{2+} channels are the main source of Ca^{2+} influx during their life cycle, obviously being adjusted to some specific patterns of activation of their functions. Thus in primary spermatocytes T-type channels are expressed in isolation and represent a primary pathway for voltage-gated Ca^{2+} entry participating in regulation of meiotic cell divison and sperm differentiation. Quite peculiarly, these channels demonstrated high sensitivity to dihydropyridines like the above mentioned LVA channels in thalamic and hypothalamic neurons (Santi *et al.* 1996). In adrenal zone glomerulosa cells secreting aldosterone this function is also triggered by minimal membrane depolarization activating dihydropyridine-sensitive LVA Ca^{2+} channels (Rossier *et al.* 1996).

The decline in the expression of LVA Ca^{2+} channels which normally takes place during cell maturation is stopped or even reversed in some pathological conditions. In pancreatic β-cells from diabetic mice macroscopic LVA Ca^{2+} currents were not present in cells from normal animals. The corresponding channels were not sensitive to classical HVA Ca^{2+}-channel inhibitors but could be blocked by amiloride and Ni^{2+}. This change might be related to the high Ca^{2+} concentration observed in β-cells during diabetes contributing to the pathogenesis of this illness (Wang, L. *et al.* 1996). A selective increase in the LVA Ca^{2+} conductance has been recorded in reticular thalamic neurons of rats with a genetic model of absence epilepsy. Whole-cell patch clamp demonstrated a substantial elevation of low-threshold Ca^{2+} currents in comparison with that in neurons of the seizure-free rat strain, retaining the usual kinetic properties, voltage dependence, and basic pharmacological sensitivity. These changes were already apparent at birth but attained significance after postnatal day 11 (again coinciding with maturation of the dendritic tree). They were quite specific for this nucleus and absent in the thalamocortical relay neurons, indicating the prominent role of LVA Ca^{2+} channels in the establishment of the thalamo–cortical synchronizing mechanisms (Tsakiridou *et al.* 1995). The prominent role of thalamic LVA Ca^{2+} channel disfunction during some form of epileptogenesis is also suggested by the data revealing the effective block of such channels by antiepileptic drugs beneficial during petit-mal seizures (ethosuximide) (Coulter *et al.* 1990). An elevation in the expression of LVA Ca^{2+} currents in thalamic (relay) neurons also has been observed in another pathologic condition—after corticotomy. One day after operation the corresponding currents became increased by 68 per cent compared with control animals. On the other hand, HVA Ca^{2+} currents did not change over the same time interval. The voltage-dependence of activation and inactivation and their time-constants remained unchanged. It has been suggested that a trophic factor is normally present which is normally retrogradely or anterogradely transported to relay neurons and acts to suppress the overexpression of T-type channels. Another possible mechanism could be a redistribution of these channels after injury due to retraction of distal dendrites, which is known to occur after axotomy, and an increase in channel density on proximal dendrites and soma (Chung *et al.* 1993). The possible functional meaning of these changes—the additional increase in $[Ca^{2+}]_i$ leading to accelerated neuronal death or, in contrast, activation of compensatory mechanisms—remains to be resolved.

The fact that in certain types of adult sensory neuron LVA Ca^{2+} channels (dihydropyridine-sensitive) also are permanently expressed can also be considered as one of the mechanisms participating in the determination of the features of their firing properties. They may be activated primarily between action potentials providing inward currents able to modulate the frequency of neuronal bursts (Ferroni *et al.* 1996).

Ontogenetic development is manifested not only in changes of the spectrum of different types of Ca^{2+} channel, but also in modifications of the membrane and intracellular mechanisms modulating their activity. It has been shown on cerebellar granule neurons growing in culture that their development is accompanied by an increase in the so called prepulse-induced facilitation—an increase in the Ca^{2+} channel current evoked by a moderate test pulse after a strong depolarizing prepulse. This facilitation may be important during the period of active synaptogenesis and is due to predominant expression of L-type channels with high unitary conductance ($\approx$25 pS) replacing channels with lower conductances (Parri and Lansman 1996). Substantial changes may also occur in the effectiveness of channel modulation by enzymatic phosphorylating systems. As has been shown in many investigations, LVA and HVA channels differ substantially in this respect, the HVA channels being subjected to extensive modulation, mainly through phosphorylation by different protein kinases, while the LVA channels are mostly insensitive to it. On peripheral (cardiac) tissues there are indications that the effectiveness and relative participation of different phosphorylating mechanisms undergo developmental changes (cf. Akita *et al.* 1994). Similar changes have been observed also in rat sensory neurons subjected to intracellular introduction of factors stimulating phosphorylation-dependent up-regulation of the activity of HVA Ca^{2+} channels (cAMP+ATP+Mg^{2+}). During intracellular dialysis of nerve cells the amplitude of HVA Ca^{2+} currents always decreases due to dephosphorylation of the corresponding channels ('run-down'). Introduction of the above mentioned factors reverses this process and restores at least temporarily the activity of Ca^{2+} channels (cf. Doroshenko *et al.* 1982). The effectiveness of such 'run-up' in rat

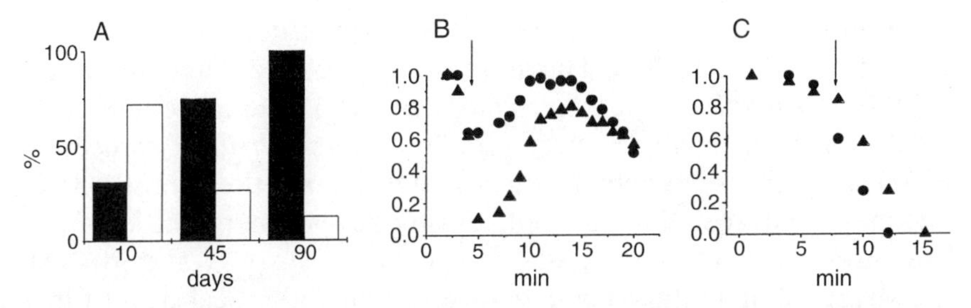

FIG 2.6 Developmental decrease in the effectiveness of up-regulation of HVA Ca^{2+} channels in rat sensory neurons. (A): developmental changes in the percentage of cells not responding (filled) and responding (open columns) to intracellular introduction of cAMP+ATP+Mg^{2+}. (B): 'run-down' of Ca^{2+} currents occurring in two neurons during cell dialysis and its reversal by introduction of the above mentioned substances (indicated by arrow). (C): absence of the up-regulatory effect in two other cells. Abscissa–time after beginning of dialysis, ordinate–normalized amplitude of Ca^{2+} currents (from Veselovsky *et al.* 1986).

sensory neurons is highly dependent on the developmental stage of the animal, being maximal in the early postnatal days and steadily declining later on.

Figure 2.6 illustrates these developmental changes in the effectiveness of metabolic modulation of HVA Ca^{2+} channels.

An interesting recent finding is that store-operated Ca^{2+} channels (SOC), known also as Ca^{2+} release-activated Ca^{2+} channels (CRAC), may be also involved in the process of neuronal differentiation. *In situ* hybridization of rat body by a cDNA clone encoding a possible candidate for CRAC on embryonic day 15 (E15) did not induce significant expression of the corresponding protein. However, on embryonic day 20 and postnatal day 1 (E20–P1) the expression signals were most evident in the septum, cerebral cortical, and hippocampal neuronal layers. Later expression again decreased (Funayama *et al.* 1996). The functional role that may be attributed to Ca^{2+} influx mediated by these channels has yet to be determined.

POTASSIUM CHANNELS

Neuronal differentiation is accompanied by a definite increase in the density of *delayed rectifier potassium channels*, their activation and deactivation becoming faster. This has been shown during *in vitro* differentiation of amphibian nerve plate and in neurons developing in culture (Barish 1986; Harris *et al.* 1988). The same holds for *rapidly inactivating potassium channels* (I_{KA}) (Desarmenien *et al.* 1993). Special changes occur in the *Ca^{2+}-activated potassium channels*: in *Xenopus* spinal neurons: they acquire their sensitivity to changes in intracellular Ca^{2+} only during development; initially they are insensitive to them in the range between 10^{-10} and 10^{-4} M. However, their unitary conductance remains identical at all times (Blair and Dionne 1985).

SODIUM CHANNELS

Sodium channels also substantially increase in density; in differentiating neuroblastoma cells this increase is especially impressive, increasing from 37.0 5.2 $\mu A\ \mu F^{-1}$ to $54.7 \pm 3.6\ \mu A\ \mu F^{-1}$ at different stages of differentiation as compared with $7.3 \pm 0.8\ \mu A\ \mu F^{-1}$ for cells in suspension (Veselovsky and Fomina 1986). It should be noted that no significant changes in the density of HVA-activated Ca^{2+} currents occur during the same developmental stages. There are indications that increased expression of sodium channels and morphological differentiation, although mostly coinciding in time, are independently regulated. Neuroblastoma cells treated with dimethyl sulphoxide (DMSO) were differentiated morphologically within 3 d, while sodium-channel expression continued to occur well after cells had assumed the morphologically differentiated state. Thus the attainment of morphological differentiation is necessary but not itself sufficient for full expression of sodium-channel proteins (Baumgold and Spector 1987). Similar progressive increases in sodium conductance occur in normal neurons in the course of their differentiation. Thus, rat immature cerebellar granule neurons displayed sodium conductances of insufficient amplitude to generate action potentials. Intermediate cells after 1–2 weeks in culture were already characterized by the presence of somatic action potentials and TTX-sensitive inward currents; longer periods of culturing were followed by loss of voltage-dependent conductances in the somatic (but not axonal) membrane. These changes may correspond to developmental changes during migration of granule neurons onto the layer of their permanent residence *in vivo* (Hockberger *et al.* 1987). In rat dorsal root ganglion neurons no substantial changes in kinetics, voltage-dependence, and density of main types of Na^+ currents were observed during the first 8 d after birth; however, changes were found in the relative amount of cells showing Na^+ currents with different characteristics: an increase in those presenting only a fast-activating TTX-sensitive channels and decrease in those representing slow, TTX-insensitive, or a mixture of both (Schwartz *et al.* 1990; Fedulova *et al.* 1994). The highly increased expression of the TTX-insensitive 'slow' Na^+ currents in rat sensory neurons during the birth period has already been demonstrated in Fig. 2.1.

In should be noted that a similar switch from expression of TTX-insensitive channels to those with high-affinity TTX sensitivity also takes place in other tissues, for instance in skeletal muscle (Haimovich *et al.* 1986) and chick heart (Kojima and Sperelakis 1985) cultures. The functional meaning of these changes is still unknown.

LIGAND-ACTIVATED CHANNELS

Glutamate-activated channels increase in density during the early stages of development. Rat cerebellar Purkinje neurons at embryonic days 20–22 (E20–22) do not respond to glutamate; a rapid increase in sensitivity takes place at postnatal days 5–9 (Hockberger *et al.* 1989). A similar increase in the density of amino acid binding sites during postnatal development occurs in cerebellar granule neurons (Cambray-Deakin *et al.* 1990). In cultured embryonic mouse hippocampal neurons responses to kainate and NMDA (glutamate, or *N*-methyl-D-aspartate) have being recorded as early as E14 and reached 100 per cent at birth (Barish and Mansdorf 1991). However, according to other sources, in mouse hippocampal neurons an increase in glutamate binding starts from postnatal day 8 and reaches a plateau at 3 weeks (Glazewski *et al.* 1993). In cultured fetal hippocampal neurons glutamate receptors became expressed 1 d after plating; later on during establishment of polarity and growth of dendrites they are first restricted to soma and dendrites and later become concentrated at the synapse-enriched portions of the dendrites, when synaptic vesicles were fully segregated to the axons. Receptor compartmentalization and dendritic redistribution took place even in the absence of externally applied glutamate and blocking of cellular activity by TTX, indicating their determination by internal developmental programming (Verderio *et al.* 1994).

A peculiar feature of developing neonatal hippocampal neurons is the synergic action of NMDA and $GABA_A$ receptors which at this time exert a depolarizing action. It has been shown on developing hypothalamic neurites that GABA can increase $[Ca^{2+}]_i$ by stimulating the cell body, resulting in an increase in calcium throughout the neuronal cell body and dendritic arbor, as well as locally, stimulating a increase in calcium only in a single dendrite or growth cone (Obrietan and Van den Pol 1996). Synaptic responses evoked by electrical stimulation of the stratum radiatum were found to be mediated by a synergistic interaction between $GABA_A$ and NMDA receptors, producing giant depolarizing postsynaptic potentials. Because of reduced voltage–dependent Mg^{2+} block of NMDA channels, substantial elevations of $[Ca^{2+}]_i$ are occurring in pyramidal neurons, which might be involved in neuronal plasticity and network formation in the developing hippocampus (Leinekugel *et al.* 1997). Later in development the role of GABA becomes more inhibitory, and glutamate plays the primary excitatory role.

Obviously, the development of glutamate-operated receptors and channels has to go in parallel with the development of corresponding *Ca^{2+} channels* responsible for the liberation of transmitter from the presynaptic terminals. A study of the role of different types of Ca^{2+} channel in transmission at the mouse neuromuscular junction has shown that after maturation the P/Q-type channels attain predominant importance. However, in newly formed junctions during reinnervation a backward shift occurs-the L-type channels became important for transmitter liberation (Katz *et al.* 1996). A study of cultured rat hippocampal neurons has shown that at least two classes of HVA Ca^{2+} channel became expressed, their relative importance changing with maturation in favour of the ω-agatoxin IVA sensitive (P-type) channel (Scholz and Miller 1995). In rat pituitary neurointermediate lobe cells during development the activity of ω-conotoxin GVIA-sensitive (N-type) and nifedipine-sensitive (L-type) channels was even observed on early postnatal days, while the activity of ω-agatoxin IVA sensitive (P-type) channels could be detected only much later (on day 42) (Beatty *et al.* 1996). A developmental redistribution of different types of HVA Ca^{2+} channels has been explicitly shown during formation of synapses between hippocampal neurons in primary culture. In parallel with increasing channel density, an enhancement of the proportion of ω-conotoxin GVIA-sensitive N-type channels at the expense of the nifedipine-sensitive L-type took place in the presynaptic structures (Basarsky *et* *al.* 1994). A similar tendency has been observed during development of rat cerebellar granule neurons in culture. A component of the KCl-depolarization-evoked Ca^{2+} entry sensitive to nifedipine (through L-type channels), and localized at cell somata, decreased with culture age. In contrast, a component blocked by ω-agatoxin IVA increased with age and whilst localized primarily at the cell somata also became evident at the neurites. This change in activity occurred at the 13th day *in vitro*. Interestingly, a Ca^{2+} entry component insensitive both to nifedipine and ω-agatoxin and localized primarily in neurites (R-type channels?) was also observed and in the early stages seemed to be involved in modulation of exocytosis. However, later (20–26th days of culture) exocytosis became sensitive mainly to ω-agatoxin and ω-conotoxin MVIIC-controlled Ca^{2+} influx (P/Q channel types) (Harrold *et al.* 1997). In PC12 cells differentiating under the influence of NGF or temperature-sensitive tyrosine-kinase, in addition to the increasing density of L- and N-type channels the P/Q-type channels also became expressed; these changes occurred without altering the channel subunit composition (Liu *et al.* 1996). A current component resistant to block by all channel antagonists (R-type?) also showed an enhanced density in differentiated PC12 cells (Lewis *et al.* 1993). The PC12 cells can also serve as a model for studying changes in channel density occurring in the opposite direction—when differentiation is stopped by chronic depolarization of their membrane (due to culturing in solution with an elevated level of K^+ ions). Under these conditions after 3 d of culturing the density of Ca^{2+} channels (measured by binding of labelled antagonists or influx of ^{45}Ca) falls by 50 per cent (DeLorme *et al.* 1988).

Ca^{2+} channels participating in synaptic transmission can be effectively modulated by chemical influences acting on definite receptors at the presynaptic membrane; down-regulation of their activity is one of the bases of presynaptic inhibition described a long time ago by Eccles and co-workers (cf. Eccles 1964). Selective adenosine (A_1) receptors exert such inhibition at excitatory hippocampal synapses. This modulatory mechanism acting mainly on N-type channels also changes in effectiveness during ontogenesis: it is much more powerful during the first two postnatal weeks (inhibiting corresponding excitatory postsynaptic currents (EPSC) by 74 ± 2 per cent) and is less effective in mature synapses (inhibition by 47 ± 3 per cent) (Scholz and Miller 1996); this will be discussed in more detail in the Chapter 3.

CONCLUSIONS

In parallel with the formation of neuronal networks, the functional properties of the elements involved show developmental changes that enable them to match their tasks. The most substantial qualitative changes occur in the population of voltage-operated Ca^{2+} channels; the LVA channels dominate in prenatal and early post-natal periods and are replaced by HVA channels later on. This specific developmental representation of LVA Ca^{2+} channels may be connected with their capability to trigger depolarization waves and intracellular Ca^{2+} transients necessary for stimulation of neuronal morphogenesis. However, in certain structures a special type of LVA channel remains well expressed during the mature state and is responsible for triggering their pacemaker activity. The spectrum of HVA Ca^{2+} channels also undergoes some developmental changes, mainly of a quantitative nature, for example a relative increase in the density of channels directly involved in synaptic transmission (N and P/Q-type). Other types of voltage- and ligand-operated channels (rapidly-inactivating, delayed rectifier, and Ca-activated K^+, TTX-sensitive Na^+, glutamate) generally show an increase in density; only the TTX-insensitive slow Na^+ channels decrease with maturation.

3

Synaptic plasticity

GENERAL FEATURES

After the formation of neuronal networks and maturation of the participating neuronal elements the main site for persistent (plastic) changes in the functioning of the nervous system becomes restricted to synaptic connections between nerve cells. Because of the extreme complexity of the mechanisms of synaptic transmission which include multiple steps of ion–protein and protein–protein interactions, this process presents huge possibilities for variations both in its effectiveness and in its time characteristics, the predominant triggering factor being changes in the firing patterns of the presynaptic elements. Plasticity of synaptic transmission has been a major topic of experimental study over the past few years, and an immense amount of data has been collected; this is often difficult to reconcile.

BASIC PHENOMENA

The basic phenomenon was first observed by Larrabee and Bronk (1947) in sympathetic ganglia and by Lloyd (1949) in the spinal monosynaptic reflex arc and designated as post-tetanic potentiation (PTP); it is manifested by an increase in the effectiveness of synaptic transmission after repetitive activation of the same synapse. Many subsequent studies have shown that the phenomenon is of general occurrence at synaptic junctions in the nervous systems of both invertebrates and vertebrates; its time characteristics are several orders of magnitude different from those of a unitary synaptic act so that it can be considered as an elementary form of plasticity retaining traces of the previous activity of the corresponding junction. Extensive analysis of PTP has shown that it is due to changes in the presynaptic structures; testing of the postsynaptic elements via presynaptic pathways other than those tetanized revealed no changes in them. The most important of these changes is a residual elevation of $[Ca^{2+}]_i$ in the presynaptic terminal, as was analysed in detail on crayfish neuromuscular junctions (Delaney *et al.* 1989; Mulkey and Zucker 1992; Kamiya and Zucker 1994) and on presynaptic terminals of mammalian cerebellar synapses (Regehr *et al.* 1994). Release of Ca^{2+} from IP_3-sensitive stores following activation of phospholipase C has also been shown to be crucially important in certain synapses (inhibitory synapses of Purkinje neurons—Hashimoto *et al.* 1996). The decay rate of the potentiated synaptic transmission resembled the decay rate of elevated $[Ca^{2+}]_i$ during the post-tetanic period. It has been concluded that the residual Ca^{2+} exerts some continuous action on sites important for the liberation of the synaptic transmitter, but different from the molecular targets triggering secretion. The interaction of Ca^{2+} with these sites may be high-affinity in nature, in contrast to processes directly involved in transmitter release (cf. Zucker 1994).

A recent finding is also the possible participation of mitochondria in synaptic PTP. Mitochondria can accumulate substantial amounts of Ca^{2+} from the cytosol due to the presence in their inner membrane of an uniporter mechanism which transports Ca^{2+} inside using the energy of the steep proton gradient always present on this membrane. Ca^{2+} can be also released back into the cytosol by Na^+/Ca^{2+} and H^+/Ca^{2+} exchangers. Ca^{2+} accumulation by mitochondria is usually considered as a low-affinity process active only when $[Ca^{2+}]_i$ levels are low. However, it has been shown recently that such accumulation takes place during physiological activity of nerve cells, diminishing the amplitudes of depolarization-induced Ca^{2+} transients due to Ca^{2+} uptake and prolonging their recovery due to slow release of ions (Kostyuk and Shmigol 1997). In parallel with these findings it has been shown on crayfish neuromuscular junctions that inhibition of mitochondrial uptake and release blocked PTP and the persistence of presynaptic residual $[Ca^{2+}]_i$ (Tang and Zucker 1997). In contrast, endoplasmic reticulum Ca^{2+}-pump inhibitors and release-channel activators had no effect. It would be quite important to test the presence of such mechanism on other synaptic junctions. The molecular receptors for this action of Ca^{2+} are still under discussion. Ca^{2+}/calmodulin-dependent protein kinase II (CaMK II) phosphorylating synapsins were considered as a likely candidates; however experiments with applications of calmodulin and CaMK kinase inhibitors were without effect on synaptic transmission and its short-term potentiation, in contrast with data about other forms of synaptic potentiation (see below). It has been shown that these mechanisms are developmentally-dependent: in chick ciliary ganglia no post-tetanic facilitation could be observed at embryonic stage E8, and a mature state was reached only at E14–15, indicating maturation of Ca^{2+} influx in the terminals and of the vesicle-associated proteins (Lin *et al.* 1996).

Plastic changes in the effectiveness of synaptic transmission attracted especial attention after the discovery in certain brain structures (hippocampus) of extremely prolonged events lasting for hours and days and designated as long-term potentiation (LTP) (Bliss and Lomo 1973). LTP became one of the most studied models of activity-evoked plasticity in the nervous system and possible basic mechanisms of information storage and memory. The problem became much more complicated after the discovery of an opposite long-lasting effect—long-term depression (LTD), manifested by stable and prolonged reduction of synaptic efficacy—which could also serve as a mechanism for introducing selectivity into neuronal pathways (Lynch *et al.* 1977; Stanton and Sejnowski 1989).

It is generally accepted that both LTP and LTD, like short-term potentiation, are closely connected with alterations in calcium signalling in the synaptic structures involved, and the discussions are focused mainly on detailed mechanisms of the action of Ca^{2+} ions. *N*-methyl-D-aspartate (NMDA) receptor activation of the corresponding type of glutamate-operated ion channels is an important factor in triggering these plastic changes because of substantial permeability of the latter to Ca^{2+} ions; the direction of changes in synaptic strength may be determined by the balance between phosphorylation and dephosphorylation of different proteins involved in the liberation of synaptic transmitters, regulated by protein kinases and phosphatases that are activated selectively by different levels of intracellular Ca^{2+} in the pre- and postsynaptic elements (cf. Debanne and Thompson 1994; Teyler *et al.* 1994).

To identify the key link in this complicated machinery, an important approach could be to simplify it and to induce artificially localized changes in calcium homeostasis. This has been done recently by injecting compounds containing caged calcium into the postsynaptic neuron and then releasing a definite amount of Ca^{2+} ions into it by photolysis (Kasono and Hirano 1995*a*; Neveu and Zucker 1996*a*, *b*). The experiments have shown that the increase of $[Ca^{2+}]_i$ in the postsynaptic cell is necessary and sufficient to induce both LTP and LTD, presynaptic activity not being obligatory for such induction. No distinctions between thresholds for these processes were detected; therefore the decision about the type of changes in synaptic efficacy probably depends on the amplitude and spread of $[Ca^{2+}]_i$ changes: for instance, to induce depression the elevation might be closer to the location of the NMDA receptors; some other as yet undetermined factor or factors may also influence the response of a cell to increased $[Ca^{2+}]_i$. Voltage-dependent differences in cytosolic Ca^{2+} acting on Ca^{2+} substrates may well occur also during natural influx of ions into the cell, compartmentalization of Ca^{2+} and its substrates aggravating such differences (Teyler *et al.* 1994). Dendritic spines can offer special possibilities for such complex interactions because of their small volume and dense packing of intracellular organelles. Model calculations of Ca^{2+} dynamics in dendritic spines taking into account intracellular Ca^{2+} stores have indicated that elevations of $[Ca^{2+}]_i$ in spines can be substantial and last for 1–2 s, thus favouring the induction of long-term changes (Schiegg *et al.* 1995).

LONG-TERM DEPRESSION

This appears to originate with smaller increases in the level of postsynaptic $[Ca^{2+}]_i$, while larger increases lead to potentiation (Lisman 1989; Artola and Singer 1993). According to the physiological mechanisms inducing such changes, LTD can be divided into two main types: activity-dependent and activity-independent. In the first case (homosynaptic or non-associative) it requires presynaptic activity in the test synaptic input (the input which subsequently exhibits LTD), in the second (which is also referred as heterosynaptic or associative) it appears in a test input after tetanization of a separate input or even antidromic activation of the postsynaptic neuron. Spread of elevated $[Ca]_i$ across the latter might be the reason for associative and heterosynaptic effects, leading to biochemical changes inducing depression of the postsynaptic effects. Low-frequency stimulation is a prerequisite for LTD; high frequencies of synaptic tetanization may trigger another biochemical pathway leading to potentiation (cf. reviews by Dudek and Bear 1992; Bear and Abraham 1996; Debanne and Thompson 1996). However, there are recent indications that this difference in the ways of triggering LTD or LTP is not a general rule and, although in hippocampal slices low-frequency stimulation usually triggers LTD, in anaesthetized or conscious rats *in vivo* it failed to induce LTD. Instead a process of erasure of long-term potentiation ('depotentiation') occurred (Doyle *et al.* 1997).

Spatial localization of the elevated $[Ca^{2+}]_i$ might also be quite important for triggering LTD; thus in cerebellar Purkinje cells LTD is connected to large but highly localized changes in postsynaptic Ca^{2+} in the finest dendritic branches induced by stimulation of the parallel fibres (Konnerth 1995). The detection of different Ca^{2+} levels in the neuron might be accomplished by different responses of protein kinases and phosphatases to Ca^{2+}. It is mostly accepted that Ca^{2+}-induced dephosphorylation of CaMK II kinase is crucial for this process (Lisman 1989; Christie *et al.* 1996) and interference with protein phosphatases blocks LTD (Mulkey *et al.* 1993; Torii *et al.* 1995), while CaMK II autophosphorylation and its conversion in a Ca^{2+} independent form favours long-term potentiation (cf. Fukunaga *et al.* 1996). Another line could be the elevated synthesis of cGMP and activation of protein kinase G (PKG). In cerebellar slices inhibition of PKG (and PKC) prevented the induction of LTD, while injection of cGMP or inhibition of its breakdown induced LTD when paired with parallel fibre stimulation. Phosphodiesterase inhibitors and 3-isobutyl-1-methylxanthine (IBMX) also induced stable LTD (Hartell 1996).

The selection of pathways for Ca^{2+} influx into the postsynaptic neuron might be also quite important for eliciting LTD. This can be VOCC located on different parts of the neuronal membrane as well as NMDA-receptor channels operated by glutamate. In an attempt to evaluate their relative importance, tetanic stimulation, which normally generates LTD in hippocampal neurons, was applied when Ca^{2+} entry via NMDA channels was limited by 2-amino-5-phosphonovaleric acid (APV) or clamping at negative membrane potentials preventing the activation of Ca^{2+} channels. However, in both cases LTD still could be induced; thus some remaining Ca^{2+} influx via either VOCC or NMDA-channels is the minimal requirement for the induction of LTD (Cummings *et al.* 1996). In neurons of rat visual cortex slices LTD could be induced after returning the slice from being kept for several minutes in elevated $[Ca^{2+}]_0$ to normal medium even when NMDA receptors were blocked; obviously, here a transient elevation of $[Ca^{2+}]_i$ through potential-dependent postsynaptic pathways is also sufficient to elicit LTD both of homo- and hetero-synaptic nature (Artola *et al.* 1996). However, many researchers have reached the conclusion that

NMDA channels are an obligatory factor in the generation of LTD (Dudek and Bear 1992; Mulkey and Malenka 1992; Izumi and Zorumski 1993; Debanne and Thompson 1994; Kasono and Hirano 1995*a*). VOCCs may be a more critical source of Ca^{2+} for induction of heterosynaptic LTD, while NMDA channels might be crucial for homosynaptic LTD (cf. review by Bear and Abraham 1996). A variety of results has been reported about the types and location of VOCC which might be involved in the generation of LTD. Some authors indicate that post-synaptic L-type Ca^{2+} channels paired with activation of metabotropic glutamate receptors are important (Bolshakov and Siegelbaum 1994). On the other hand, there are indications that induction of LTD in the hippocampus can be blocked by Ni^{2+} but not by nimodipine, indicating possible participation of LVA (T-type) Ca^{2+} channels (Wang, Y. *et al.* 1996).

The release of Ca^{2+} from intracellular stores may also play an important role in triggering LTD. In cultured Purkinje neurons heparin injcctions (blocking the $InsP_3$-gated release of Ca^{2+}) prevented the induction of LTD by coupling glutamate application and depolarization. In contrast, liberation of caged $InsP_3$ in conjunction with depolarization induced LTD (Kasano and Hirano 1995*b*). In hippocampal slices both thapsigargin and cyclopiazonic acid—compounds that deplete all intracellular Ca^{2+} pools by blocking ATP-dependent Ca^{2+} uptake—blocked the induction but not the maintenance of LTD without affecting baseline synaptic transmission; thus release of Ca^{2+} from presumably $InsP_3$-gated stores might be required for such induction. Bath application of ryanodine, inducing selective depletion of the ryanodine receptor-gated Ca^{2+} pool also blocked the induction of LTD; however, no such block appeared if ryanodine was introduced in the postsynaptic neuron through a microelectrode. This may indicate that ryanodine-sensitive stores involved in the induction of LTD are located in presynaptic elements (Reyes and Stanton 1996).

It has to be mentioned that long-lasting depression in hippocampal neurons can also be evoked by direct stimulation with transmembrane current stimuli; such depression outlasts stimulation by up to 170 s and is functionally very similar to trans-synaptically evoked LTD. However, such depression is due to activity-dependent modifications in intrinsic properties of the stimulated cells, with little if any synaptic participation. Possible reasons suggested for this depression are a gradual decline in the speed at which Ca^{2+} is buffered intracellularly and a corresponding increase in the slow

Ca^{2+}dependent potassium current ($I_{K(Ca)S}$) activation rate (Borde *et al.* 1995).

The question about the possible presynaptic expression of LTD is still under discussion. Data show that in hippocampus the depression is connected not only to a decrease in postsynaptic responses to glutamate, but also to a long-term decrease in transmitter release from presynaptic terminals (Bolshakov and Siegelbaum 1994). In this case the question arises about a possible retrograde messenger triggering changes in the presynaptic structures. Nitric oxide has been suggested as a candidate, because, according to some data, its inhibitors block LTD induced by low-frequency afferent stimulation in rat hippocampus (Izumi and Zorumski 1993). From experiments on rat cerebellar Purkinje neurons it has been concluded that nitric oxide-donors induce their effect at both presynaptic and post-synaptic sites. The presynaptic depression fades away with wash-out of nitric oxide-donors and may be mediated through potentiation of A_1-adenosine receptors (see below). Part of this effect may be due to non-nitric oxide products. LTD expressed at a postsynaptic site may be directly induced by nitric oxide, is independent on the ADP ribosylation, and involves mainly the production of cGMP (Blond *et al.* 1997). However, some authors did not find any effect of NO donors on LTD (Cummings *et al.* 1994; Malen and Chapman 1997).

Long-term depression of synaptic transmission is obviously a basic phenomenon present not only in highly developed nervous systems but also in its lower forms. Thus it appears in sensorimotor synapses from *Aplysia* activated by prolonged low-frequency stimulation of the sensory neuron. As in mammals, its induction can be blocked by infusion of Ca^{2+} buffers (BAPTA) into the postsynaptic cell (Lin and Glanzman 1996).

It can be concluded that a number of key issues still need to be resolved before definite conclusions can be drawn as to the involvement of any specific routes of Ca^{2+} entry in LTD (cf. Christie *et al.* 1996).

LONG-TERM POTENTIATION

This involves much more obvious functional changes in the presynaptic structures of the synaptic junctions, although the initial trigger in this case is also an elevation of intracellular Ca^{2+}. The quantal analysis of changes in excitatory post-synaptic potentials

(EPSPs) and results obtained by a variety of other approaches indicate that at least the initial stages of LTP are predominantly of presynaptic origin, manifested by an increase in probability of transmitter release from both high- and low-efficacy release sites in activated synaptic terminals (cf. review by Voronin 1993) . Figure 3.1 illustrates these increases manifested by changes of EPSPs recorded from a hippocampal CA1 neuron.

As in the case of LTD, LTP can be divided into subtypes depending on the mechanisms of induction of the initial elevation of intracellular Ca^{2+}. The most studied type of potentiation is that occurring in hippocampal neurons. In the pyramidal cell it can be induced by stimulation of two different synaptic inputs: axons of granule cells (mossy fibres) which terminate on proximal dendrites of pyramidal cells, and associational/commisural (Schaffer) collaterals (SCC) forming synapses on the rest of the dendritic tree. In the second case the synapses are similar to the excitatory synapses found on dentate granule cells and are associated with high levels of NMDA receptors; thus long-term changes in their efficacy are entirely dependent on the activation of the latter. This type of synaptic transmission is predominant in pyramidal neurons of the CA1 hippocampal region. In contrast, mossy fibre synapses, predominant in the CA3 region, are associated with a low level of NMDA receptors and repetitive activation of these synapses results in an NMDA-independent form of LTP (Harris and Cotman 1986). Similarly, plasticity of excitatory synaptic transmission in neocortical (visual) neurons is also not dependent on NMDA receptors, and VOCCs are responsible for supply of Ca^{2+} ions (Komatsu 1994).

In the case of *NMDA-dependent forms of LTP* the NMDA-receptor channels should be the main source of elevated Ca^{2+} in the postsynaptic cell necessary for triggering all subsequent events (cf. Perkel *et al.* 1993). However, the situation here is obviously not so simple, and additional mechanisms are likely to be involved to make this process effective. In the experiments of Malenka *et al.* (1992) on activation of a photolabile Ca^{2+} buffer in a CA1 hippocampal neuron at specific periods of LTP development it was shown that intracellular $[Ca^{2+}]_i$ has to be elevated for a considerable time (longer than 1.5 s) to be able to trigger LTP. This cannot be achieved simply by activation of NMDA channels, and VOCC also must participate. Both components are attenuated by inhibition of CaM kinase (Huber *et al.* 1995). It has been shown on hippocampal neurons that inhibition of Ca^{2+}-dependent protein phosphatase 2B (calcineurin)

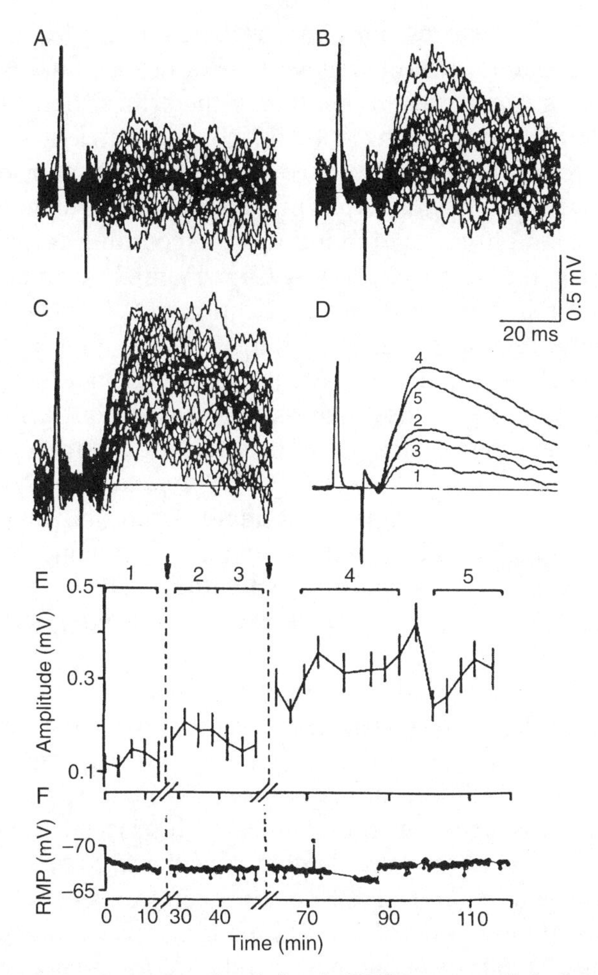

FIG 3.1 Quantal changes of minimal EPSPs recorded from a CA1 hippocampal neuron during LTP induced by tetanic stimulation of Schaffer collaterals. (A–C): single EPSPs before (A) and after tetanization which produced smaller (B) and larger (C) LTP. (D–E): superimposition of averaged control (1) and post-tetanic (2–5) EPSPs recorded at different time intervals after tetanus. (F): resting membrane potential of the neuron in the same experiment (from Voronin 1993).

by okadaic acid supports the activity of VOCCs, relieving them from tonic dephosphorylation ('run-up') (Mironov and Lux 1991). Therefore somewhat surprising are recent findings that inhibition of calcineurin in apical dendrites of CA1 hippocampal neurons, which might support the activity of Ca^{2+} channels, prevented the induction of LTP (Wang and Stelzer 1994). It has also been suggested that if intracellular Ca^{2+} stores and Ca^{2+} release in dendritic spines are taken into account, sustained elevations of intracellular Ca^{2+} can be predicted to be necessary to overcome the critical period necessary for LTP induction (Schiegg *et al.* 1995). In any case, extracellular Ca^{2+} is required during the whole period of induction of LTP; its removal even 15–30 min after burst stimulation significantly decreased the amplitude of potentiation. According to some recent observations, the activity of HVA Ca^{2+} channels seemed not to be important for such support, but application of Cd^{2+} or Ni^{2+} inhibited it, indicating possible participation of LVA (T-type) channels (Katsuki *et al.* 1997). In contrast, in rat striatal neurons long-term enhancement of the release of dopamine, resembling LTP, has been found to depend on the activity of L-type Ca^{2+} channels (Koizumi *et al.* 1995).

Activation of metabotropic glutamate receptors (mGluRs) also seems to be involved in the induction and maintenance of LTP; the possible mode of action could be activation of PKC regulating the function of NMDA receptors (see review by Riedel and Reymann 1996).

As the NMDA-dependent form of LTP is critically dependent on Ca^{2+} influx in the postsynaptic neuron and at the same time is based on long-lasting changes in the functioning of presynaptic elements, an important and still disputed question is the nature of the possible retrograde messenger which combines both processes. Arachidonic acid and its metabolites were the first considered to be implicated in retrograde signalling during LTP as they can freely pass through cell membranes (Collingridge 1987). Later nitric oxide was considered by many investigators as the main candidate for such a role (Bashir and Collingridge 1992; Snyder 1992; Jessel and Kandel 1993; Malen and Chapman 1997). However, the induction of LTP in CA1 neurons could not always be blocked by inhibitors of NO production (Gribkoff and Lum-Ragan 1992); therefore other substances can be also considered as such messengers (see below).

The intracellular events responsible for long-lasting modulation of the functioning of presynaptic terminals during LTP may include several signalling pathways, which in turn may act on different steps in the mechanism of Ca^{2+}-triggered exocytosis. One includes the already mentioned CaM-kinase II and Ca^{2+}-dependent phosphatase (calcineurin). Both calmodulin and the two enzymes are highly concentrated in nerve terminals; the activated kinase phosphorylates synapsin I which may induce cytoskeletal rearrangements and changes in transmitter-release parameters. In contrast, activation of calcineurin will eliminate the auto-phosphorylation of CaM kinase and therefore play a role in the limitation of LTP. Another pathway that may potentiate presynaptic secretion can act through metabotropic activation of PKC. PKC can modulate the presynaptic output–input relations via several mechanisms, which include direct modulation of the activity of K^+ and Ca^{2+} channels, modulation of transmitter production as well as recruitment, docking, and release of synaptic vesicles. The activation of adenylyl cyclases and cAMP-dependent protein kinases may also be required for late stages of LTP, acting in synergism with other CaM-sensitive cyclases (Xia *et al.* 1995). A detailed analysis of the extremely complicated multistep process of Ca^{2+}-dependent exocytosis has been given in several reviews (Augustine *et al.* 1994; Verhage *et al.* 1994).

The structural and functional changes in the presynaptic structures have not yet been precisely defined. An important component which has recently been directly visualized is an increase in the exocytotic–endocytotic cycling rate measured by uptake of antibodies which recognize the intraluminal domain of the synaptic vesicle protein synaptotagmin (Malgaroli *et al.* 1995). The degree of potentiation was heterogeneous, appearing greater at synapses at which the initial extent of vesicular turnover was low. Another important finding is the demonstration of the involvement of new NMDA synapses in the potentiated synaptic transmission. It has been shown that in hippocampal CA1 neurons under an increased external Ca^{2+}/Mg^{2+} ratio the stimulation of Schaffer collaterals induces a substantial prolongation of excitatory postsynaptic currents due to a dramatically increased contribution of its NMDA-dependent component, indicating the existence of silent NMDA-receptors or even synapses in this system (Klishin *et al.* 1994, 1995*b*; Lozovaya and Klee 1995). A factor which promotes such change is the blockade of A_1-adenosine receptors which when active are able to suppress excitatory synaptic transmission via G-protein-mediated feed-back mechanisms (see below). A similar effect could be produced by application of phorbol esters activating PKC by mimicking the action of the physiological activator diacylglycerol and probably disrupting G-protein-mediated adenosine inhibition (Schwartz 1993).

This new component disappeared under application of either NMDA or non-NMDA antagonists, indicating that involvement of additional NMDA receptors or synapses is mediated by a complicated, probably polysynaptic, pathway. Figures 3.2 and 3.3 present

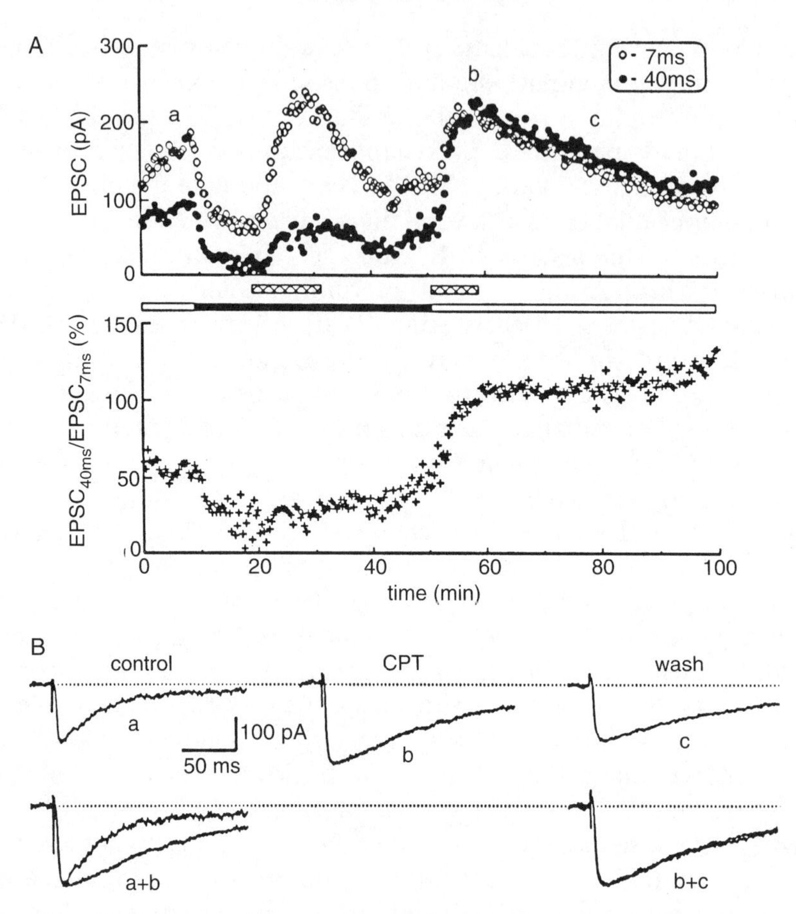

FIG 3.2 Facilitatory effect of A_1-receptor blockade by CPT on EPSCs in hippocampal CA1 pyramidal neuron. A–changes in EPSC amplitudes measured 7 and 40 ms after stimulation; B–examples of EPSC records in control, after CPT application and its wash-out. Filled bars in A indicate external standard solution, open bars indicate solution with elevated Ca^{2+}/Mg^{2+} content, and hatched bars indicate application of 250 nM CPT (from Klishin *et al.* 1995*a*).

examples of the described changes recorded in CA1 rat pyramidal hippocampal neurons in slices. Figure 3.2 illustrates the effectiveness of potentiation of EPSC after blocking the A_1 receptors by use of 8-cyclopentyltheophylline (CPT), and Fig.3.3 the extreme stimulus-dependent prolongation of EPSC which was triggered by stimulation of SCC pathways in the presence of CPT (record 2) as well as the NMDA-receptor antagonist 2-amino-5-phosphonovaleric acid (APV) (record 3), and again became evident after its removal (record 4).

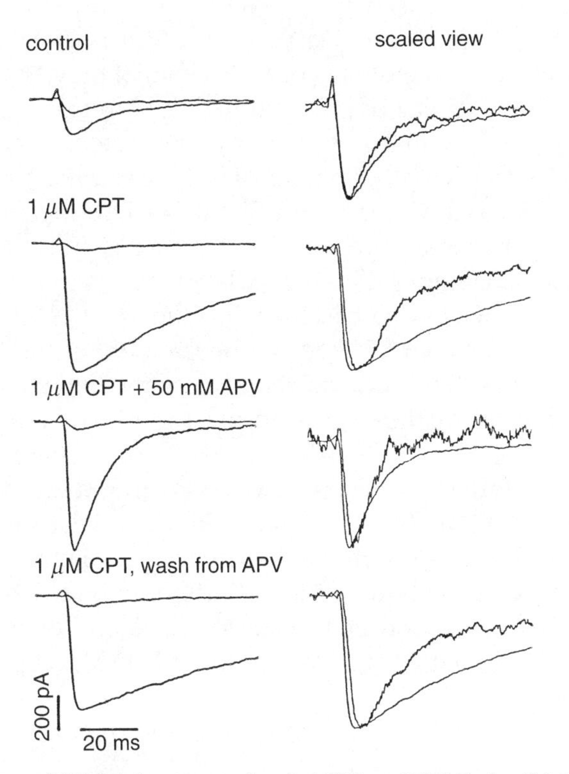

FIG 3.3 Effect of NMDA antagonist d-APV on EPSCs in CA1 pyramidal neuron previously modified by CPT. The traces were obtained at two different stimulus strength and normalized in the right column. APV blocks the action of CPT on the prolonged stimulus-dependent component of EPSC, but it became evident again after APV washout (Klishin *et al.* unpublished data).

It has been suggested that after Schaffer collaterals repeatedly excite CA1 neurons via predominantly non-NMDA-receptor-mediated synapses, the pyramidal neurons start to excite each other recurrently via the normally silent NMDA-receptor-mediated synapses (see Fig. 3.4). This leads to prolonged enhancement of their activity, which persists at least 2 h after removal of the adenosine-receptor antagonist (Klishin *et al.* 1995*a*). Thus, a powerful system of NMDA-receptor-mediated synaptic contacts may exist around the hippocampal pyramidal neurons which is silent at rest due to tonic presynaptic inhibition via A_1 receptors, but becomes released when this activity is blocked. A rapidly diffusing factor released by the stimulated axons could be responsible for such a block. An investigation of the role of this inhibition in the modulation of different types of VOCC has shown that 40–50 per cent of it is directed to N-type channels, although other types of Ca^{2+} channel may also participate. In addition, the efficacy of presynaptic inhibition has been found to decline with synapse maturation, partly because of a developmental decline in the relative contribution of N-type channels to transmitter release (Scholz and Miller 1996). Silent NMDA-mediated synaptic contacts may become activated also during ischaemia, which can induce post-ischaemic LTP. It has been shown that after even a single episode of transient ischaemia numerous NMDA-receptor-mediated synaptic contacts became operational in the CA1 area of the hippocampus. Thus anoxia seems to some extent to be equivalent to inhibition of the A_1-adenosine receptors (Tsintsadze *et al.* 1996)

The involvement of silent NMDA-operated synapses in the generation of LTP in the CA1 hippocampus has also been suggested by Malinow *et al.* (1995). In whole-cell voltage-clamp investigations of pyramidal cells dialysed with Ca buffers failures of postsynaptic responses were recorded in a hyperpolarized and depolarized state of the cell; in the latter case (when the NMDA-receptor-mediated

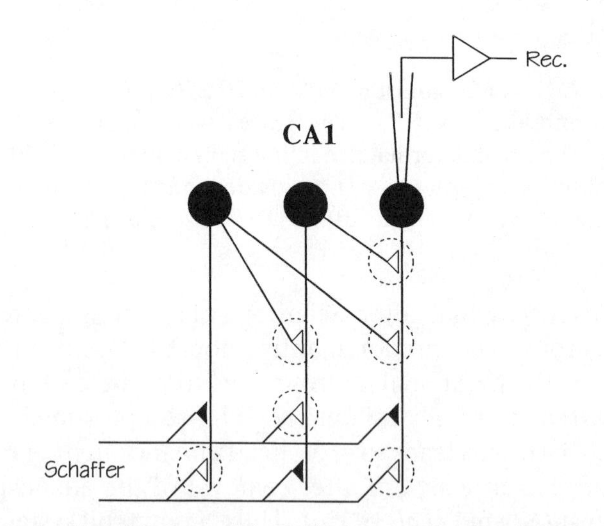

FIG 3.4 Simplified model of CA1 synaptic circuitry that may account for the activation of latent synaptic interconnections. Filled synaptic terminals (triangles) represent Schaffer collateral excitatory input with both NMDA and non-NMDA components to CA1 pyramidal neurons (circles) and open synaptic terminals—NMDA-receptor-mediated connections. Broken circles indicate initially silent synapses that are recruited after blocking A_1-receptors.

synapses were released from Mg^{2+} block) the number of failures decreased more then twofold, obviously indicating the transition of some from a silent to an active state. After blocking the NMDA receptors by APV this difference disappeared, and the number of failures became the same as in hyperpolarized condition. A Monte Carlo simulation of the effects of inclusion of new synapses into the generation of LTP has been conducted (Malinow and Mainen 1996), however, alternative explanations of these results were presented by others.

The NMDA-independent form of LTP induced by mossy fibre stimulation differs from the previously described form in many respects. Its induction in the CA3 hippocampal region remained essentially normal when synaptic transmission was blocked by glutamate receptor antagonists, but ceased in the absence of extracellular Ca^{2+}. This indicates that *presynaptic* Ca^{2+} entry may be essential for triggering this form of synaptic plasticity (Castillo *et al.* 1994). Attempts were made to determine the type of VOCCs important for such entry. Postsynaptic responses induced by mossy fibre stimulation were little affected by blocking the L-type Ca^{2+} channels, partly inhibited by blocking N-type, and almost completely inhibited by blocking P-type channels. However, none of these interventions alone prevented mossy-fibre LTP. Thus its development is not critically connected to activation of a certain type of presynaptic Ca^{2+} channel, and Ca^{2+} ions required for its induction can enter through any of them. When their concentration in the terminal rises to a critical level, it triggers a series of events downstream from Ca^{2+} entry which increase the sensitivity of the transmitter release mechanism to Ca^{2+}.

It should be kept in mind that in the CA3 region the mossy fibres also activate a substantial NMDA receptor synaptic component (Weisskopf and Nicoll 1995). The question arises why do mossy fibres here not express NMDA-receptor-dependent LTP? Experiments with the use-dependent NMDA receptor antagonist MK-801 have indicated that the probability of transmitter release remains enhanced during the expression of mossy fibre LTP, indicating that both induction and expression of LTP here are presynaptic. A conclusion can be drawn from these results that the molecular machinery responsible for NMDA-dependent LTP is absent in these synapses.

An important question is whether the NMDA-independent form of LTP might occur at other synapses except those between mossy fibres and CA3 hippocampal pyramidal cells. A recent publication confirmed that a similar type of LTP develops at synapses between parallel fibres and Purkinje neurons in the cerebellum (Salin *et al.* 1996). Repetitive stimulation of parallel fibres in a cerebellar slice caused a long-lasting increase in synaptic strength, associated with a decrease in paired-pulse facilitation. Blockade of glutamate receptors did not prevent LTP induction, nor did loading of Purkinje neurons with a Ca^{2+} chelator. LTP was occluded by forskolin-induced activation of adenylyl cyclase and blocked by protein kinase A inhibitors. These findings suggest that parallel fibre synapses express a form of LTP that is dependent on the activation of a presynaptic adenylyl cyclase and is indistinguishable from LTP at hippocampal mossy fibre synapses. It remains to be determined if this enhancement is due to upregulation of presynaptic VOCCs or to some steps subsequent to the entry of Ca^{2+} into the presynaptic terminals.

In thc hippocampal dcntate gyrus LTP of field EPSPs was induced by high-frequency stimulation of the medial perforant-granule cell pathway and LTD by low-frequency stimulation; in this case mGluRII receptor agonists strongly inhibited the induction of LTP, while their antagonists reverted this block, at the same time inhibiting the induction of LTD (Huang *et al.* 1997). It has been suggested that in this system LTP induction is also connected with an increase in presynaptic cAMP concentration, perhaps via an increase in intracellular Ca^{2+} level, activation of mGluRII receptors inhibiting such increase. In contrast, LTD induction may be inhibited by such a rise in cAMP; thus an antagonistic action on mGluRs will inhibit the induction of LTD.

An important question is the possible participation of other neurotransmitters in the induction of non-NMDA forms of LTP. In the case of LTP evoked in the hippocampal dentate gyrus from the perforant path it has been shown that propranolol, a β-adrenoreceptor antagonist, blocked LTP induction of both lateral and medial perforant path-evoked field EPSPs (Bramham *et al.* 1997). This may indicate a broad requirement for norepinephrine in synaptic plasticity at least in certain types of synaptic connection.

Long-term potentiation in the visual and frontal cortex evoked by stimulation of the white matter also requires the activation of NMDA receptors. In most neurons, the presence of bicuculline was required for the induction of LTP, indicating that the threshold of an NMDA receptor is strongly influenced by inhibitory processes (cf.

review by Kaczmarek *et al.* 1997). However, a special type of NMDA-independent LTP has been recorded in neurons of kitten visual cortex. Here LTP could be induced by low-frequency conditioning stimulation of the white matter in the presence of NMDA antagonist APV; such stimulation failed to induce LTP when activation of LVA Ca^{2+} channels was prevented either by membrane depolarization or by bath application of 100 μM Ni^{2+} . When cells were impaired by an electrode containing Ca-chelator (BAPTA), LTP was never induced; thus Ca^{2+} influx into the postsynaptic cell is in this case critical for such induction (Komatsu and Iwakiri 1992). A definite developmental dependence of this form of LTP should be noted: it was maximal at the critical period of visual cortical plasticity (fifth week after birth) and almost disappeared in adult animals.

Obviously, the induction of LTP should also be NMDA-independent in the case of synapses using other kinds of transmitter, for instance inhibitory transmitters. In fact it has recently been shown that LTP can develop in visual cortical inhibitory (GABAergic) synapses on layer V cells in conditions when the ionotropic glutamate receptors were blocked. LTP induction could be prevented by the application of $GABA_A$, but not by $GABA_B$ or metabotropic glutamate receptor antagonists. Elevation of $[Ca^{2+}]_i$ in the postsynaptic cell was a prerequisite for the induction of LTP, as in the above mentioned case, while buffering intracellular Ca^{2+} with low-affinity buffer resulted in a marked inhibition of inhibitory postsynaptic currents (IPSCs). However, the main source of Ca^{2+} here was its liberation from IP_3-sensitive stores and not influx through VOCCs, as LTP could be induced during clamping of the membrane at various voltages between –90 and +20 mV, but was prevented by loading them with the $InsP_3$-receptor antagonist heparin or emptying stores by addition of caffeine (De Koninck and Mody 1996). Induction of LTP could be also facilitated by the activation of α_1-adreno- and 5-HT_2 receptors, all acting through some G-protein-coupled intracellular pathway (Komatsu 1996). A interesting speculation can be made from these data about the functional significance of LTP mediated by the inhibitory connections in the visual cortex. Because the *locus coeruleus* and *raphe* nucleus cells—the sources of catecholamines and serotonin in the cortex—maintain high activity during periods of wakefulness but not during sleep, potentiation of inhibitory synapses might occur just when the animal is looking attentively at its visual environment, obviously increasing its discriminative capability.

In other brain structures an opposite effect may occur during the development of a special form of LTP—*long-term synaptic disinhibition* (for example impairment of the function of inhibitory synapses). In CA1 hippocampal neurons the inhibitory responses in their apical dendrites became enhanced shortly after tetanic stimulation of Schaffer collaterals, the enhancement later being replaced by depression. Similar depression was observed in responses to iontophoretically applied $GABA_B$ receptor agonists. Disinhibition was dependent on elevation of $[Ca^{2+}]_i$ in the postsynaptic cell and could be prevented by the same interventions which prevented the induction of NMDA-dependent LTP of excitatory synaptic connections, indicating the existence of shared cellular pathways in the induction of LTP and synaptic disinhibition (Wang and Stelzer 1996). A special investigation of EPSPs in inhibitory interneurons during stimulation of Schaffer collaterals which induces LTP in pyramidal cells has shown that excitatory synapses onto interneurons undergo a long-term synaptic depression ('interneuron LTD'—iLTD). Unlike other forms of hippocampal synaptic plasticity, iLTD is not synapse specific: stimulation of an afferent pathway triggered depression not only of activated synapses but also of inactive excitatory synapses onto the same interneuron (McMahon and Kauer 1997). These data suggest that high-frequency afferent activity may increase hippocampal excitability through a dual mechanism, simultaneously potentiating synapses onto excitatory neurons and depressing synapses onto inhibitory ones. However, the question about the interrelations of possible post- and presynaptic changes during disinhibition remains open.

Synaptic disinhibition has also been analysed in another structure—cerebellar Purkinje neurons. Depolarizing trains applied to these neurons induce in them a transient decrease of inhibitory transmitter (GABA) release. The effect is dependent on postsynaptic rise of $[Ca^{2+}]_i$ and includes two components. One is manifested by a decrease in the rate of miniature IPSCs, another also involves modulation of the excitability of the presynaptic endings and can be transmitted along the presynaptic axon and modify the activity of its arborizations on other postsynaptic cells (Glitsch *et al.* 1996). It has been found that the effect can be mimicked by a specific agonist of group II mGluRs and inhibited by drugs which interfere with these receptors. It has been suggested that here glutamate or glutamate-like substances liberated from the postsynaptic cell in response to elevated $[Ca^{2+}]_i$ act as the retrograde messenger acting on presynaptic mGluRs, which in turn are negatively coupled to adenylate cyclase. A decrease of the cAMP level in presynaptic terminals in some way attenuates the release of inhibitory transmitter. This suggestion is supported by the finding that application of forskolin, which increased the cAMP level, reduced disinhibition, and increased synaptic activity. The results may also offer a new candidate for the position of retrograde messenger in hippocampal long-term potentiation and disinhibition.

LONG-TERM FACILITATION IN INVERTEBRATES

As in the case of long-term depression, long-term facilitation of synaptic transmission phylogenetically is also an ancient phenomenon, forming the basis of learning in invertebrates, although its molecular mechanisms may be different from those in mammals. Heterosynaptic long-lasting facilitation of transmission following presynaptic activation of a facilitatory (modulatory) presynaptic pathway observed in mollusc ganglia has been considered to depend on changes in presynaptic transmitter release, postsynaptic activation being neither sufficient nor necessary for its induction. Activation of serotoninergic neurons may be important for producing these changes. 5-HT has been shown to produce long-lasting changes in the functioning of molluscan neurons. They include persistent modulation of the activity of different types of ion channel mediated by different intracellular messenger systems. A special type of 5-HT-sensitive K^+ current called S-current has been found to decrease in *Aplysia* neurons under the action of 5-HT due to phosphorylation-dependent closure of the corresponding channels; this leads to broadening of the action potentials and enhancement of transmitter release, as well as to increased axonal firing (Klein *et al.* 1986; Siegelbaum *et al.* 1986). The activity of several other types of potassium channel (I_{KA} and $I_{K(Ca)}$) also becomes down-regulated via a specific G-protein which may be phosphorylated by PKC and CaM kinase II (Nelson *et al.* 1990); similar multiple inhibitory effects were observed in *Helix pomatia* neurons, but one type of K^+ channel here proved to be stimulated by 5-HT (Lukyanetz and Sotkis 1996*b*).

In contrast, the activity of Ca^{2+} channels becomes up-regulated by 5-HT. A comparison of the effects induced in the same cell by application of 5-HT or by elevation of the intracellular cAMP level in different ways has shown their non-additivity, confirming the

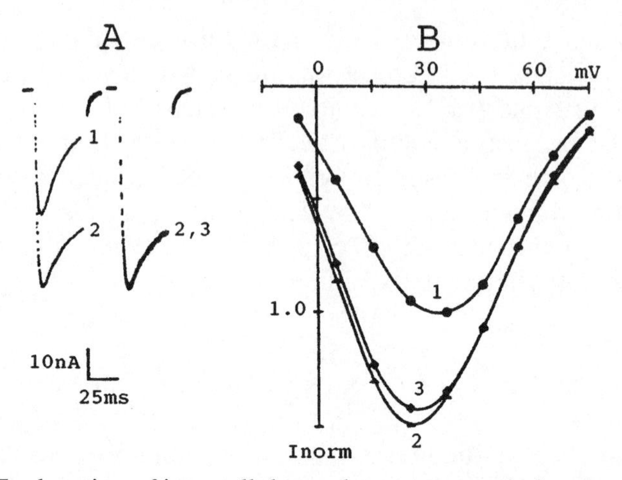

FIG 3.5 Exploration of intracellular pathways up-regulating the activity of neuronal Ca^{2+} channels by serotonin in the snail *Helix pomatia.* Records of currents are presented in control (1), after application of 5-HT alone (2), and in combination with injection of cAMP or the catalytic subunit (CS) of protein kinase A (3). No additivity of the combined effects is observed indicating that the action of 5-HT is entirely mediated through cAMP-mediated phosphorylation of Ca^{2+} channels (from Kostyuk *et al.* 1992).

conclusion that the action of 5-HT is mediated through cAMP-dependent phosphorylation (or inhibition of dephosphorylation by Ca-dependent phosphatase) (Kostyuk *et al.* 1992). Figure 3.5 illustrates the effectiveness of this cAMP-mediated up-regulatory action of 5-HT on Ca^{2+} currents in an identified *Helix* neuron. It should be mentioned that VOCCs in molluscan neurons cannot be directly compared with those in mammals. Although resembling HVA channels by their activation characteristics, they have a low unitary conductance (like that of LVA channels) and weak specificity to typical Ca^{2+} channel antagonists.

In this case a switch to down-regulation may occur if the rise of $[Ca^{2+}]_i$ becomes excessive, leading to Ca^{2+}-calmodulin-dependent activation of phosphodiesterase and phosphatase, preventing Ca^{2+} channels from being phosphorylated (Kostyuk and Lukyanetz 1993, 1994). As these enzymatic mechanisms show different sensitivity to intracellular Ca^{2+}, a complicated concentration dependence appears for the down-regulatory process. First, only Ca^{2+}-dependent phosphodiesterase becomes activated due to its low K_d value which stops further up-regulation of Ca^{2+} channels. However, if $[Ca^{2+}]_i$ continues to rise, active dephosphorylation of Ca^{2+} channels by

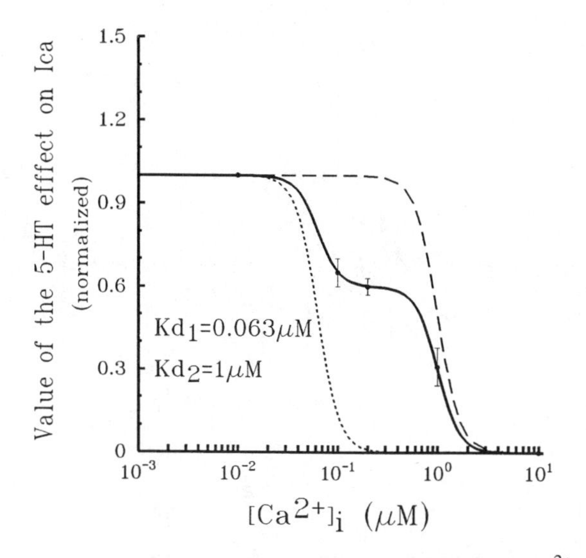

FIG 3.6 Curtailing of the up-regulatory effect of 5-HT on Ca^{2+} channels in *Helix* neurons by excessive elevation of intracellular Ca^{2+} level. The normalized up-regulated amplitude of Ca^{2+} currents is plotted against $[Ca^{2+}]_i$ level changed by intracellular injections of Ca^{2+} buffer. The results are fitted by a binding isotherm with two different K_d values, indicating the participation of two different Ca^{2+}-dependent enzymes (from Kostyuk and Lukyanetz 1993).

calcineurin begins (Kostyuk and Lukyanetz 1993, 1994, see Fig. 3.6).

Analysis of the level of single-channel activity has shown that 5-HT prolongs the mean open time of Ca^{2+} channels and proportionately decreases their mean closed times; it also evokes an increase in the number of active channels. All the effects illustrated in Fig. 3.7 are exerted on the channels indirectly via intracellular messenger systems, as they appear during addition of 5-HT to the bath solution without direct contact with the membrane fragment (Lukyanetz and Sotkis 1996*a*).

The role of 5-HT in the induction of long-lasting facilitation of synaptic transmission has been tested directly on monosynaptic connections between sensory and motor neurons of *Aplysia* in culture; here 5-HT could induce both short-term and long-term facilitation depending on the number of 5-HT applications. The short-term effect could be triggered by direct action of 5-HT on the mechanism of transmitter release, the long-lasting one by new protein synthesis triggered by phosphorylation of transcription-

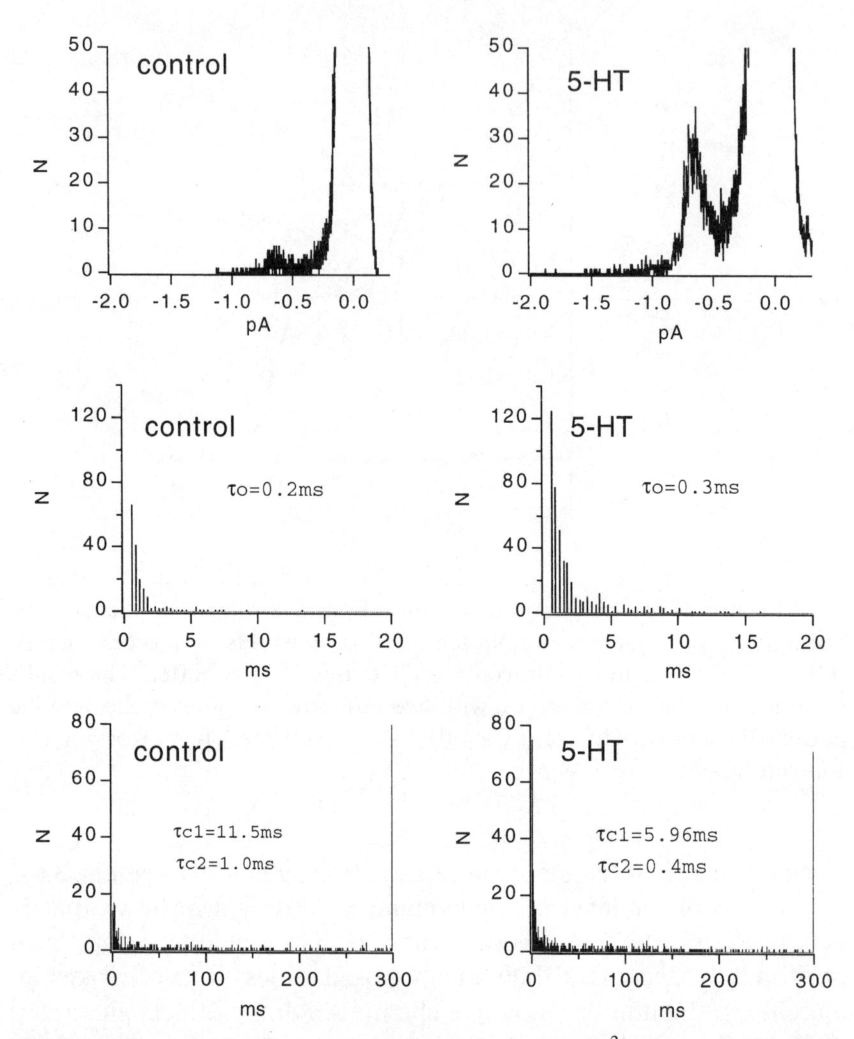

FIG 3.7 Changes in the functioning of single Ca^{2+} channels in *Helix* neurons under the action of serotonin. (A): amplitude histograms indicating an increase in number of active channels with unitary currents about 0.7 pA. (B): open and closed time histograms indicating prolongation of open times (τ_o) and shortening of closed times (τ_{c1} and τ_{c2}). (From Lukyanetz and Sotkis 1996*a*).

activating proteins. Single exposures to 5-HT (or cAMP as the second messenger for 5-HT) led to phosphorylation of several substrate proteins that was not dependent on transcription or translation, while repeated or prolonged exposure to these factors induced long-term changes in phosphorylation of the same proteins dependent for their induction on both translation and transcription (Sweatt and Kandel 1989). Newly synthesized proteins could be used for structural changes at activated postsynaptic sites or secreted as extracellular signals leading to changes in presynaptic transmitter release (Mauelshagen *et al.* 1996) .

The powerful capability of 5-HT to induce plastic changes in invertebrate synaptic junctions may stimulate a more detailed analysis of the possible role of 5-HT in the induction of plastic changes in the functioning of mammalian synapses.

It should be noted that in *Aplysia* sensorimotor synapses the induction of long-term facilitation, like LTP in mammalian synapses, can be regulated by postsynaptic voltage (Lin and Glanzman 1996). In *Helix* ganglia LTP also could be induced by tetanic stimulation of the postsynaptic neuron with concomitant presynaptic activation, probably involving increased postsynaptic Ca^{2+} and some retrograde messenger (Bravarenko *et al.* 1995).

CONCLUSIONS

Long-term changes in the effectiveness of synaptic connections is the main form of plasticity in the mature nervous system. They can be manifested both in facilitation and depression of synaptic transmission and can affect both excitatory and inhibitory synapses in vertebrates as well as invertebrates, although their expression is quite variable in different structures. Transient elevation of intracellular Ca^{2+} induced in the presynaptic terminals or postsynaptic neurons by repetitive firing of the afferent fibres is the main natural trigger of these changes; in the latter case some retrograde messenger is required to induce parallel changes in the presynaptic elements. Long-term changes in the effectiveness of transmitter liberation is the most evident mechanism of synaptic plasticity; however, more profound changes may also be involved in the form of activation of silent receptors or even synapses. The intracellular pathways linking Ca^{2+} transients with these functional changes are still not completely analysed; they may affect existing proteins involved in synaptic transmission via their phosphorylation or dephosphorylation by different Ca^{2+}- and calmodulin-dependent protein kinases and phosphatases, as well as synthesis of new proteins via induction of both transcription and translation.

4

Aging and neuronal functions

GENERAL FEATURES

Changes in neuronal functions with aging are well known from everyday life; they can in general be considered as negatively-directed neuronal plasticity and include loss of neuronal elements and functional changes in those surviving. There are numerous data indicating that alterations in Ca^{2+} homeostasis in nerve cells may be of crucial importance in brain aging and age-dependent deficits in its functions, similarly to their crucial role in the formation of neuronal networks. A large variety of experiments has already been performed to characterize alterations of Ca^{2+}-regulating mechanisms with aging. They include investigations of general changes in intracellular Ca^{2+} level in aged cells, alterations in the functioning of Ca^{2+} channels, Ca^{2+} stores, and extrusion mechanisms, and especially changes in the functioning of synaptic connections.

RESTING LEVEL OF FREE CA^{2+} IN AGED NEURONS

Obviously, this question has to be asked first in attempts to clarify the mechanisms of age-related changes of neuronal functions. However, the answers given by different authors are quite contradictory. According to Hartmann *et al.* (1993*a*), the basal level of $[Ca^{2+}]_i$ is significantly reduced in mechanically dissociated neurons from aged mice. It has been suggested that the reduced basal level of $[Ca^{2+}]_i$ makes the Ca^{2+}-dependent intracellular process more sensitive to Ca^{2+} during aging (Hartmann *et al.* 1994). Later on these authors described region-specific features of this decline: it was substantial in neurons from the hippocampus and neocortex, but not in those from the striatum or cerebellum (Hartmann *et al.* 1996*a*, *b*).

In contrast, an *increase* in cytosolic free Ca^{2+} with age was found in rat brain synaptosomes (Martinez-Serrano *et al.* 1988, 1992;

Satrustegui *et al.* 1996). The reason for this was a reduction of binding capacity of the cytosolic compartment (excluding mitochondria and endoplasmic reticulum). Das and Ghosh (1996) also found in uptake experiments an increased plasma content of $^{45}Ca^{2+}$ in rat cortex and hippocampus only. In our experiments a substantial elevation of resting $[Ca^{2+}]_i$ was observed in cultured primary sensory neurons isolated from old rats as compared with those from adult animals (207 ± 37 nM versus 96 ± 23 nM—Kirischuk *et al.* 1992). A similar difference was found in cerebellar granule neurons recorded in slices from old and adult rats (Kirischuk *et al.* 1996*c*). In sympathetic ganglion neurons the difference was 92 ± 13 nM versus 60 ± 9 nM (Duckles *et al.* 1996). Figure 4.1 presents statistical data from our group about the resting levels of $[Ca^{2+}]_i$ in rat primary sensory, hippocampal, and neocortical pyramidal neurons as compared with those in neurons from newborn and adult animals.

There is an obvious explanation of such an increase—the reduction of Ca^{2+} efflux from the cells because of decreased activity of Na^+/Ca^{2+} exchanger and plasmalemmal Ca^{2+}–ATPase (PMCA pump), as well as loss of cytosolic Ca-binding proteins, although data about such losses in different animal species and different structures are extremely variable. Loss of calbindin and calretinin with aging

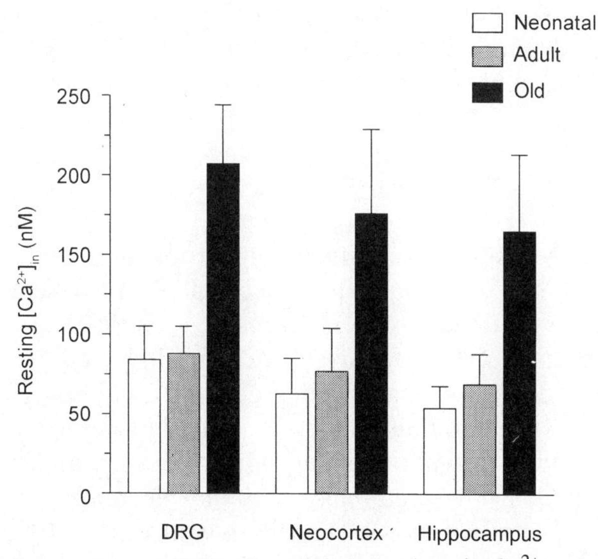

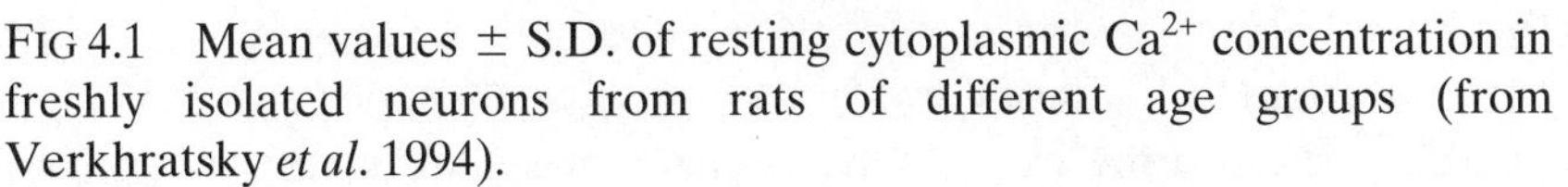
FIG 4.1 Mean values ± S.D. of resting cytoplasmic Ca^{2+} concentration in freshly isolated neurons from rats of different age groups (from Verkhratsky *et al.* 1994).

was observed in rat hippocampus, but not in cerebellum, by Villa *et al.* (1994). In rat retina calbindin was found to decrease progressively with aging, while calretinin remained unchanged; no changes in calbindin were found in cortical area (Papazafiri *et al.* 1995). Immunoreactivity for calbindin was found to be dramatically reduced in aged rat hippocampal neurons; the same was found for immunoreactivity for parvalbumin in the cingulate cortex and medial septal area by Krzywkowski *et al.* (1996), whereas no change was observed for calretinin. Age-related loss of calbindin in rat hippocampus was also observed by De Jong *et al.* (1996); a peculiar finding was the absence of calbindin-immunoreactivity in the same structures even in young rabbits, which makes a causal role of calbindin changes in functional decline of hippocampal neurons somewhat doubtful. An age-related decrease in mitochondrial Ca^{2+} uptake was observed in rat brain synaptosomes (Martinez-Serrano *et al.* 1992; Satrustegui *et al.* 1996); impairment in the activity of the calcium uniporter appears to underlie this defect.

The functional implications of these changes in the basal level of intracellular Ca^{2+} are not clear; obviously, they may render aged cells more sensitive to damaging influences which by themselves act by filling them with excessive amounts of Ca^{2+}. They could affect also the characteristics of Ca^{2+} transients during neuronal activity. Therefore substantial efforts have been made by many authors to evaluate age-dependent changes in characteristics of Ca^{2+} transients; however, data about such changes are also quite controversial.

AGE-DEPENDENT CHANGES IN CA^{2+} TRANSIENTS

In our experiments on rat and mice dorsal root ganglion neurons we found a substantial *decrease* in the density of HVA Ca^{2+} currents and corresponding reduction of Ca^{2+} transients (Kostyuk *et al.* 1993; Verkhratsky *et al.* 1994, cf. review by Kirischuk and Verkhratsky 1996). Typical examples of such a decrease of $[Ca^{2+}]_i$ transients in rat sensory and neocortical neurons are presented in Fig. 4.2. Figure 4.3. presents statistical data about changes in the density and availability of Ca^{2+} channels in these animals. A similar decrease was found in hippocampal granule neurons (Reynolds and Carlen 1989) and, in the periphery, in colonic smooth muscle cells (Xiong *et al.* 1993). Measurements of radioligand binding in aged Fischer rats revealed decrease in 1,4-dihydropyridine density in striatum, hippocampus,

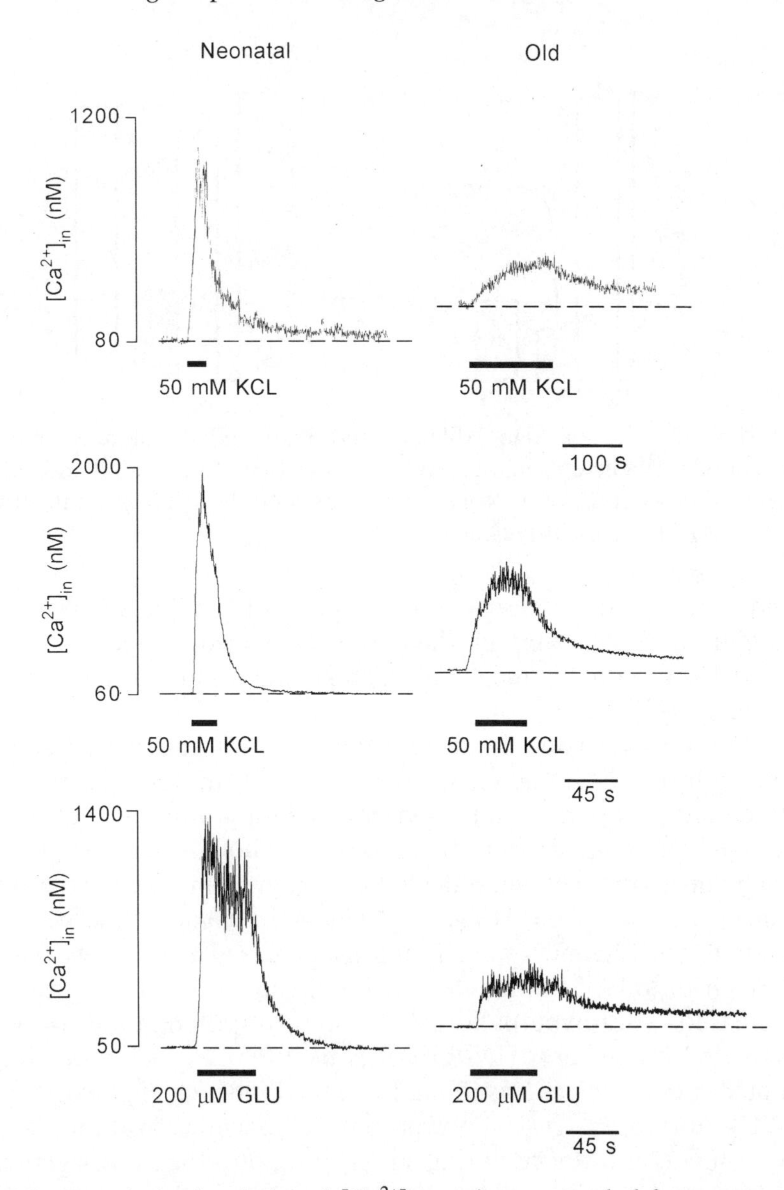

FIG 4.2 Depolarization-induced $[Ca^{2+}]_i$ transients recorded from sensory (A) and neocortical (B) neurons of newborn and old rats. Cell depolarization was induced by application of high-K^+ solution (A, B) or 200 μM glutamate (from Verkhratsky *et al.* 1994).

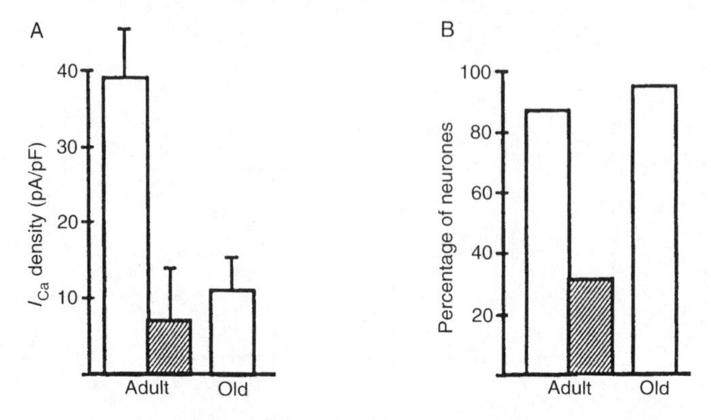

FIG 4.3 Density of high- (blank) and low- (filled columns) voltage-activated Ca^{2+} currents in rat DRG neurons isolated from adult and old rats (A) and percentage of neurons which expressed these components of Ca^{2+} currents (B) (from Kostyuk *et al.* 1993).

and cortex and a decrease in ω-conotoxin binding in the hippocampus and striatum; in the latter case also a decrease in K^+ depolarization-mediated $^{45}Ca^{2+}$ uptake was found (Bangalore and Triggle 1995).

On the other hand, in an extensive series of papers by Landfield and colleagues an age-dependent *increase* in Ca^{2+} current was described in brain (mainly pyramidal hippocampal) neurons (cf. review by Landfield 1996). It was observed both in cultured neurons and neurons in slices and reflected a substantial increase in density of functionally available HVA Ca^{2+} channels (Campbell *et al.* 1996); even T-type channels were found in increased density (Murchison and Griffith 1995; Thibault and Landfield 1996). There was also increased after-hyperpolarization due to potentiation of Ca^{2+}-activated K^+ currents (Disterhoft *et al.* 1996). A factor which promoted these changes was found to be the influence of glucocorticoid (GC) hormones. It is known that excessive activation of GC-receptors (for instance during stress) promotes the brain-aging processes, and a possible mechanism could be the corresponding alterations in Ca^{2+} homeostasis (Kerr *et al.* 1992; Landfield *et al.* 1992). These changes were also considered as a factor in the increased vulnerability of aged neurons, being inversely correlated with the learning ability of aged animals.

In peripheral neurons the opposite changes were also reported by different investigators. Thus, norepinephrine release from cardiac synaptosomes induced by K^+ was reduced in aged rats due to reduction of Ca^{2+} movement (Snyder *et al.* 1995), while in the tail artery of the same animal it increased with advancing age, due probably to elevated cytosolic Ca^{2+} and its inhibited mitochondrial uptake (Buchholz *et al.* 1994; Tsai *et al.* 1995).

Definitely, the modulation of the activity of Ca^{2+} channels by their enzymatic phosphorylation or dephosphorylation also changes in effectiveness during aging. In our experiments on DRG neurons from young and old rats this has been demonstrated by comparing the effects of neuronal dialysis and introduction of substances involved in channel-protein phosphorylation. It is known that wash-out of soluble components from the cytosol during intracellular dialysis leads to the disappearance of the metabolic support of HVA Ca^{2+} channels and a progressive decrease ('wash-out') of the corresponding I_{Ca}. As has been shown in Chapter 2, this decrease can be slowed or even reversed by the addition of cAMP+ATP to the intracellular solution. We found that metabolic dependence of HVA I_{Ca}, very pronounced in neurons from newborn and adult animals, became insignificant in neurons obtained from old ones. Moreover, the run-down of I_{Ca} became definitely slower in old neurons. The results are illustrated on Fig. 4.4 where the run-down of I_{Ca} measured in the presence or absence of cAMP and ATP in the intracellular solution is compared. Mean run-down half-life was practically unaffected by cAMP and ATP in aged neurons, whereas it was clearly slower in young ones (Verkhratsky *et al.* 1994). Thus HVA Ca^{2+} channels in old neurons seem to loose the capability to be regulated by cytoplasmic phosphorylation.

While data about age-dependent changes in the amplitude of Ca^{2+} currents in different neuronal structures are quite controversial, data about the time-course of these currents and the corresponding intracellular Ca^{2+} transients are more consistent—prolongation of both characteristics with aging has been generally observed. Substantial prolongation of Ca^{2+} spikes has been described in rat hippocampal slice neurons (Pitler and Landsfield 1990) which were followed by prolonged Ca^{2+} transients; extremely prolonged $[Ca^{2+}]_i$ transients were directly measured in rat primary sensory neurons (Verkhratsky *et al.* 1994). This has already been illustrated in Fig. 4.2, and Fig. 4.5 presents statistical data about changes in the half-life of the decay of depolarization-induced $[Ca^{2+}]_i$ transients in primary sensory, pyramidal neocortical, and hippocampal neurons from old animals. Several mechanisms could be responsible for such changes. On one hand, they could be due to changes in the regulation of Ca^{2+}

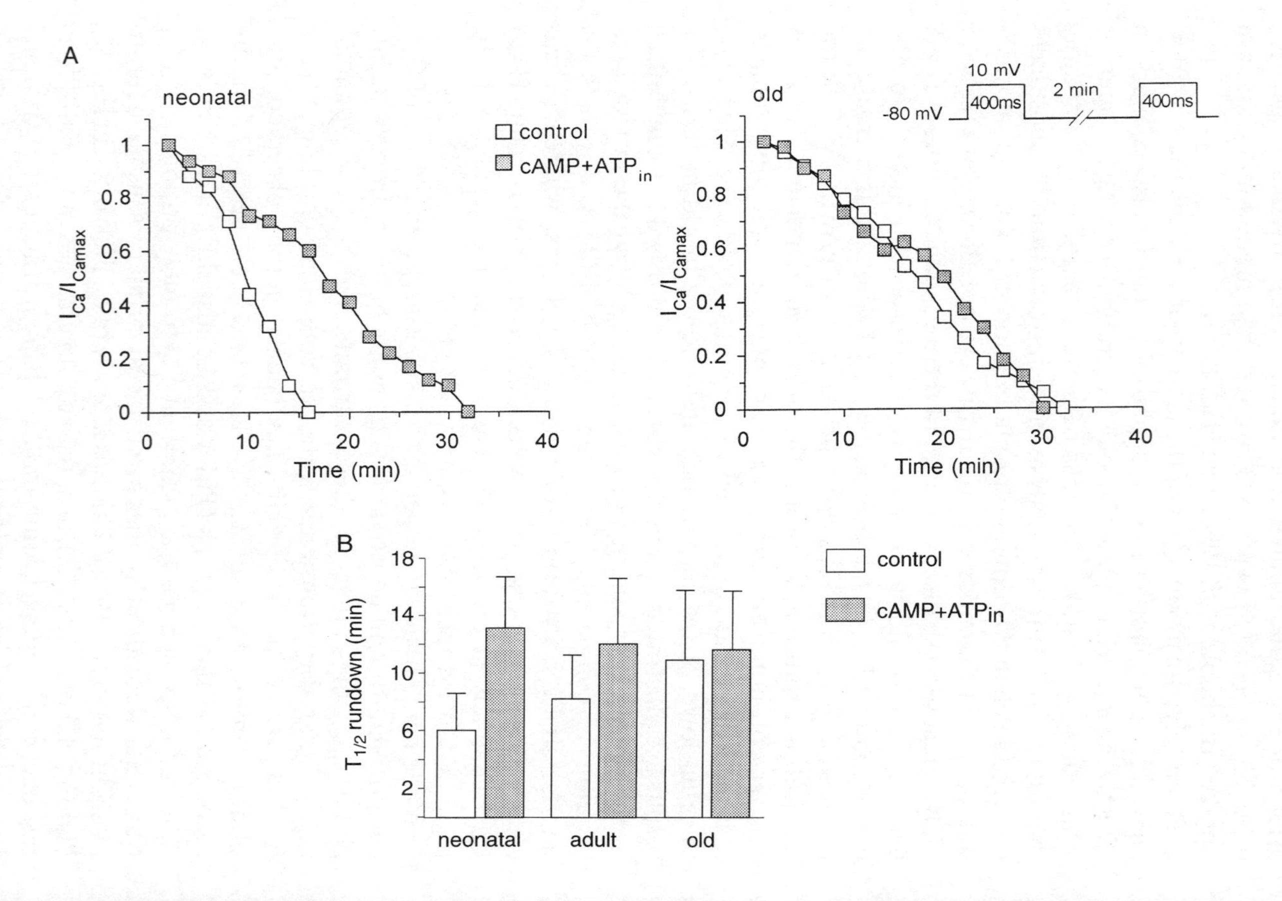
A
neonatal
control
cAMP+ATP$_{in}$
I_{Ca}/I_{Camax}
Time (min)
old
10 mV
-80 mV
400ms
2 min
400ms
B
$T_{1/2}$ rundown (min)
neonatal
adult
old

FIG 4.4 Run-down of HVA Ca^{2+} currents and effect of intracellular administration of cAMP+ATP in rat DRG neurons form newborn, adult, and old rats. (A): comparison of run-down of I_{Ca} recorded in the absence and presence of cAMP+ATP in the intracellular perfusion solution (pulse protocol is presented on the inset). (B): Statistical data about the dependence of the run-down half-life from the presence of cAMP+ATP in the intracellular solution (from Verkhratsky *et al.* 1994).

channels (slow-down in inactivation); there was significantly less slow inactivation in aged basal forebrain neurons (Murchison and Griffith 1996), although in DRG sensory neurons we did not observe substantial changes in inactivation kinetics. On the other hand, alteration of the mechanisms responsible for removal of excessive Ca^{2+} from the cytosol (accumulation by the endoplasmic reticulum and extrusion through plasmalemmal mechanisms) were also found. CaM-activated PMCA pump activity was found to decrease with age, particularly when CaM isolated from aged animals was used to stimulate the enzyme (Michaelis, 1994; Michaelis *et al.* 1996), the intracellular stores in sensory neurons became overfilled with Ca^{2+} (judging by the amplitudes of transients which could be induced by activation of CICR by caffeine) and probably less capable of accumulating excessive Ca^{2+} from the cytosol (Kirischuk *et al.* 1992; Verkhratsky *et al.* 1994) and so Ca^{2+}-stimulated inositol phosphate hydrolysis increased (Hartmann *et al.* 1994). Changes in mitochondrial Ca^{2+} uptake have already been mentioned.

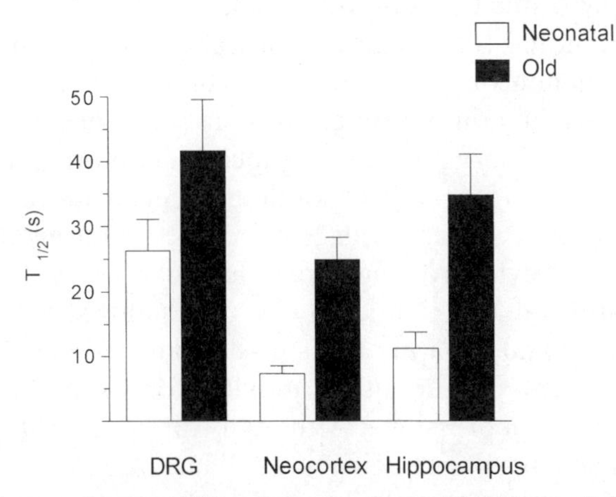

FIG 4.5 Mean values ± S.D. of the recovery half-lives of depolarization-induced $[Ca^{2+}]_i$ transients in rat sensory and central neurons obtained from neonatal and old rats (from Verkhratsky *et al.* 1994).

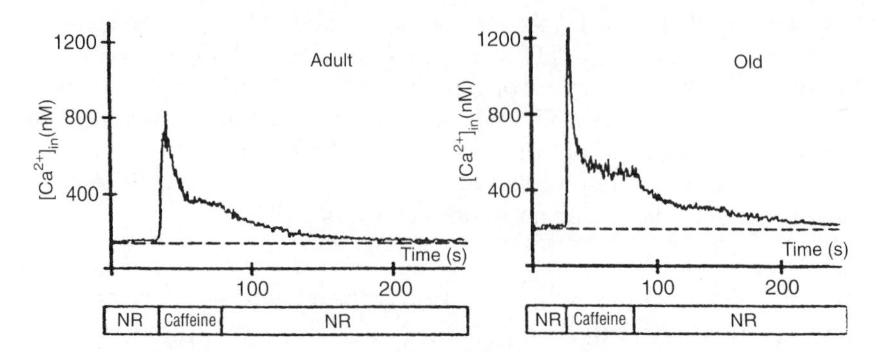

FIG 4.6 Caffeine-induced $[Ca^{2+}]_i$ transients in DRG neurons from adult (A) and old (B) rats (from Kirischuk *et al.* 1992).

Figure 4.6 presents records of caffeine-induced $[Ca^{2+}]_i$ transients in rat DRG ncurons from adult (A) and old (B) rats. As can be seen from the records, these neurons are capable of accumulating in their stores and releasing substantial amounts of Ca^{2+} at rest, but during aging this amount becomes substantially higher. Central neurons (for instance, neocortical and hippocampal pyramidal cells) normally do not hold many Ca^{2+} ions in their stores at rest, but effectively accumulate them if the Ca^{2+} level in the cytosol is increased (see Fig. 4.7A). But during aging their stores also became constantly filled with Ca^{2+} and cannot be charged further even after substantial elevations of cytosolic Ca^{2+} (Fig. 4.7B, C).

It should be noted that changes in intracellular Ca^{2+} homeostasis demonstrated in neuronal cells are to a certain extent mirrored (or at least paralleled) in non-neuronal cells, for instance lymphocytes. Consistent with observations of reduced depolarization-induced Ca^{2+} increase in neurons, corresponding reduced mitogen-induced Ca^{2+} responses were observed in lymphocytes from aged mice and circulating lymphocytes from aged people (Eckert *et al.* 1994)

Such alterations in the kinetics of Ca^{2+} transients should definitely impair interneuronal synaptic transmission and especially its components dependent on repetitive activity, for example long-term potentiation and depression. Although direct investigations of corresponding changes with aging are still lacking, there is a general belief that they could create the basis of senile changes in perception and learning.

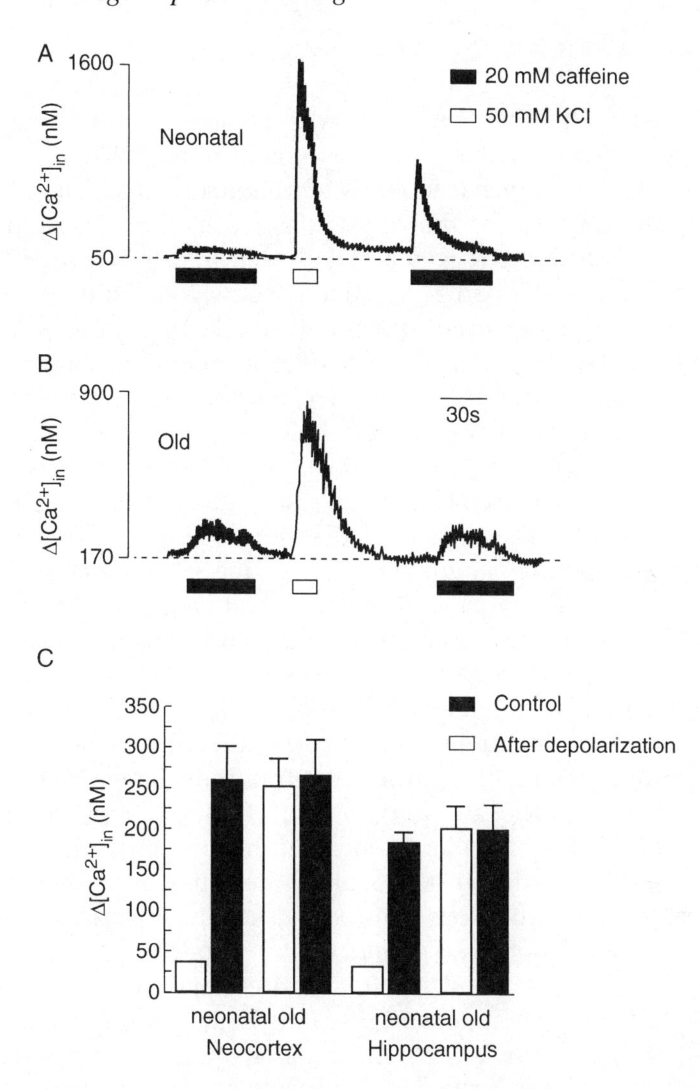

FIG 4.7 Caffeine-induced $[Ca^{2+}]_i$ transients in rat brain neurons from neonatal (A) and old (B) rats. Transients in hippocampal neurons were compared before and after charging the neuronal stores by elevation of cytosolic Ca^{2+} (via high K^+-induced membrane depolarization). (C) presents mean amplitudes ± S.E. of such transients recorded in neocortical and hippocampal pyramidal neurons (from Verkhratsky *et al.* 1994).

NEURONAL DEGENERATION AND DEATH

As has been already been mentioned, age-dependent alterations in Ca^{2+} homeostasis make aged cells much more sensitive to pathological situations which frequently terminate in cell degeneration and death. Among them the most dangerous are ischaemia and Alzheimer's disease. It is widely believed that in both cases intraneuronal Ca^{2+} overload is the main factor contributing to neurodegeneration. However, the magnitude of Ca^{2+} accumulation, and its duration and segregation within distinct intraneuronal compartments may contribute differently to the incidence of degenerative processes in different neuronal systems. Another variable is the type of Ca^{2+}-dependent enzymes and protein–protein interactions which might be activated. The increased $[Ca^{2+}]_i$ can result from influx of calcium from the extracellular space, from redistribution of intracellular stores or from both sources coupled by Ca^{2+}-induced Ca^{2+} release (CICR). A variety of effects can follow such disregulation. They include activation of proteases, endonucleases, and phospholipases, all of which can contribute to the cellular changes that occur during the prelethal phase (cf. reviews by Trump and Berezesky 1995, 1996).

It should be mentioned that before the development of deep changes in cellular metabolism, more transient changes may occur in membrane properties under the effect of oxygen deprivation. They are manifested by hypoxic membrane hyperpolarization, which is associated with reduced neuronal input. It has been shown on rat hippocampal CA1 neurons *in vivo* that such hyperpolarization is due to activation of both K_{ATP}- and Ca^{2+}-dependent K^+ channels, the release of Ca^{2+} from intracellular stores, and activation of CaM kinase II playing an important role in such activation (Yamamoto *et al.* 1997). Therefore potassium-channel openers (bimakalim) are able to maintain neuronal viability after chemical anoxia, while ATP-sensitive potassium-channel blockers (tolbutamide) reverse this protective action; protection is due to inhibition of neurotransmitter release, as it does not work in case of direct glutamate-induced neurotoxicity (Wind *et al.* 1997).

It seems that later one of the most important Ca^{2+}-regulated processes contributing to ischaemia-evoked neurodegeneration is the Ca^{2+}-dependent cysteine protease calpain I (μ-calpain). Calpain I is half-maximally activated by 3–20 μM $[Ca^{2+}]_i$, therefore under normal conditions it is largely inactive. However, in cultured neurons where $[Ca^{2+}]_i$ has been assessed directly, either anoxia or treatment with excitatory amino acids evoking delayed Ca^{2+}-dependent degeneration raised the $[Ca^{2+}]_i$ level above 1 μM, sufficient to lead to activation of calpain I (cf. Siman *et al.* 1996). This activation is accompanied by the degeneration of neuronal structural proteins that are preferred calpain substrates. Several neuronal populations, including pyramidal neurons of the hippocampal CA1 area, show especially marked calpain-degraded products. On the other hand, calpain inhibitors are neuroprotective by influencing processes that occur subsequent to the ischaemic insult. At the same time, some hippocampal neurons that do not exhibit a rapid calpain activation in response to ischaemia still go on to die. In this case delayed and sustained calpain activation was correlated with neuronal vulnerability; thus a protracted $[Ca^{2+}]_i$ rise may play a more important role in delayed neuronal death. Measurements on hippocampal neurons in culture have shown that the time required for the recovery of $[Ca^{2+}]_i$ from the increased level after exposure to glutamate to pre-stimulus levels closely paralleled the degree of neuronal loss, resembling the delayed type of cell death (Ogura *et al.* 1988). However, despite all these convincing data, it should be kept in mind that calpain activation may be controlled not only by the magnitude and duration of the rise of intracellular Ca^{2+} but also by other factors. The extent to which $[Ca^{2+}]_i$ is elevated may also not absolutely determine the severity of the toxic insult. Local transients or sustained low-level augmentations may be equally effective events (cf. Dubinsky 1993). The degree of mitochondrial participation in the sequestration of Ca^{2+} entering the cell could be also quite important. If this mechanism is not damaged, the destructive changes in the cell may be delayed by many hours; this may be one of the reasons for differences in Ca^{2+}-related cell death *in vivo* and *in vitro* (Kristian *et al.* 1996). On the other hand, there are data indicating that in certain cases mitochondrial Ca^{2+} accumulation may be a *necessary* intermediate in excitotoxicity—if a cellular microdomain below the plasmalemma is accessible to mitochondria and they can rapidly accumulate Ca^{2+} from this domain, thus removing feed-back inhibition of NMDA receptors by intracellular Ca^{2+} and increasing overflow of Ca^{2+} into the cell through NMDA-activated channels (Budd and Nicholls 1996). This Ca^{2+} accumulating function of mitochondria is, of course, quite limited. During Ca^{2+} uptake the membrane potential of the mitochondria decreases, the extent of the decrease being proportional to the amount of Ca^{2+} taken up; finally their membrane potential would collapse.

One of the early signs of the activation of proteases are perturbations of cytoskeletal organization and interconnections between the plasmalemma and cytoskeleton. They include modifications of the association between actin and actin-binding proteins and proteolysis of the latter, disruption of microtubular organization; appearance of multiple surface protrusions ('blebs'). Altered balance of protein kinase/protein phosphatase activity may result in abnormal phosphorylation of cytoskeletal and other proteins finally leading to cell death (cf. review by Orrenius *et al.* 1996). It should be mentioned that necrotic cell death in adult life may be not the only outcome; apoptosis which is the mechanism of programmed death during fetal development has been demonstrated also in certain disease conditions. The changes included activation of Ca^{2+}-dependent endonucleases, resulting in cleavage of cell chromatin, compacting of organelles, widespread plasma and nuclear membrane blebbing, etc. Interestingly in many cells the initial Ca^{2+} increase was found in the nucleus, suggesting that a selective elevation of the nuclear Ca^{2+} concentration may be sufficient to stimulate DNA fragmentation. The enhanced Ca^{2+} influx through excessive stimulation of amino acid-receptor-operated membrane channels appears to play an important role in neuronal damage; there is evidence that NMDA receptor/channel blockers blocked DNA degradation and apoptosis in cerebellar granule cells (Orrenius *et al.* 1996). However, this conclusion seems to be not always true. In some studies it has been shown that elevation of cytosolic Ca^{2+} could block apoptosis (Franklin and Johnson, 1994). Obviously, further studies are required to define the role and mechanisms of Ca^{2+}-mediated neuronal death.

Another potential mechanism of Ca^{2+}-triggered neurotoxicity which has been discovered is represented by nitric oxide (NO) synthase. It has been suggested that the generation of NO triggered by $[Ca^{2+}]_i$ increase caused by glutamate-receptor over-stimulation of NO synthase-containing neurons may be lethal to neighbouring cells by inducing DNA damage. The NO synthase-containing neurons themselves seem to be less sensitive to NO toxicity (Dawson *et al.* 1991). Recent direct investigations of the influence of prolonged action of nitric oxide on hippocampal neurons in culture have shown persistent alterations in Ca^{2+} homeostasis, especially in recovery kinetics of $[Ca^{2+}]_i$ transients induced by membrane depolarization, indicating probable impairment of Ca^{2+} removal from the cytoplasm (Brorson *et al.* 1997).

Ca^{2+} overloading is the initial damaging step during Alzheimer's disease and several other neurodegenerative diseases. Deposition of β-amyloid peptides (Aβ), consisting of 39–42 amino acids, is one of the causal agents of Alzheimer's pathology. They insert themselves into plasmalemma and form ionic channels also permeable to Ca^{2+} (cf. Arispe *et al.* 1994). Therefore neurons exposed to Aβ show a dramatic rise of $[Ca^{2+}]_i$; this rise may be the direct reason for neuronal degeneration or a signal making them more susceptible to other pathogenic influences like aging. In dissociated neurons from adult mice preincubation with β-amyloid fragment 25–35 resulted in a 100% amplification of the K^+-induced $[Ca^{2+}]_i$ response, the effect already being seen at very low peptide concentrations (50 nmol L^{-1}) and occurring within minutes (Hartmann *et al.* 1993). Epidemiological studies have indicated that the incidence of Alzheimer's dementia starts to increase exponentially after the age of 65, indicating that age-dependent and Alzheimer's-dependent Ca^{2+} overload potentiate each other in their deleterious effects (cf. Disterhoft *et al.* 1994; Winiewski and Frangione 1996).

The leading hypothesis for neuronal death during another neurodegenerative disease—amyotrophic lateral sclerosis—is also excitotoxic damage and Ca^{2+} overload; however, an autoimmune basis has also been considered suggesting the existence of antibodies to Ca^{2+} channels leading to increased channel open-time and increased Ca^{2+} influx. Immunoglobulin preparations from ill patients were shown to induce death of a rat motoneuron/mouse neuroblastoma cell line, and the effects were prevented by blockade of N- or P-type Ca^{2+} channels (Smith *et al.* 1994). However, recently some doubts were expressed about the mechanism of action of such immune preparations and possible contamination of the effect by proteolytic activity, so the question has to be re-examined (cf. Vincent and Drachman 1996).

Some common features can be found in the mechanisms of brain aging and neurodegenerative disorders during diabetic neuropathy, as has been emphasized in a review by Biessels and Gispen (1996). Disturbed calcium homeostasis is one of important features during diabetic complications. They can be the result of ischaemia, oxidative stress and non-enzymatic glycosylation accompanying diabetic hyperglycaemia. In experiments on mice with streptosotozin (STZ)-induced or genetically determined insulin-dependent diabetes we have found substantial alterations in intracellular Ca^{2+} homeostasis in certain types of nerve cell, especially in small-size primary sensory cells transmitting nociceptive signals. These cells differ from large-size neurons transmitting propioceptive signals by the absence of functional Ca^{2+} stores accumulating excessive Ca^{2+} from the cytosol; therefore Ca^{2+} extrusion from these neurons is exerted almost exclusively by the plasmalemmal Ca pump (PMCA) (Shmigol *et al.* 1995*b*). Non-enzymatic glycosylation during chronic hyperglycaemia may predominantly affect just plasmalemmal proteins; PMCA being one of those specifically depressed (cf. Vlassara *et al.* 1994). Therefore Ca^{2+} homeostasis becomes substantially altered specifically in nociceptive cells; the time course of $[Ca^{2+}]_i$ transients being extremely prolonged, resembling in this respect the changes in Ca^{2+} signalling in aged neurons already described (Kostyuk, E. and Shmigol 1995*a*; Kostyuk, E. *et al.* 1995). Typical examples of the described prolongation of calcium signals in nociceptive neurons of mice with experimental diabetes are presented in Fig. 4.8.

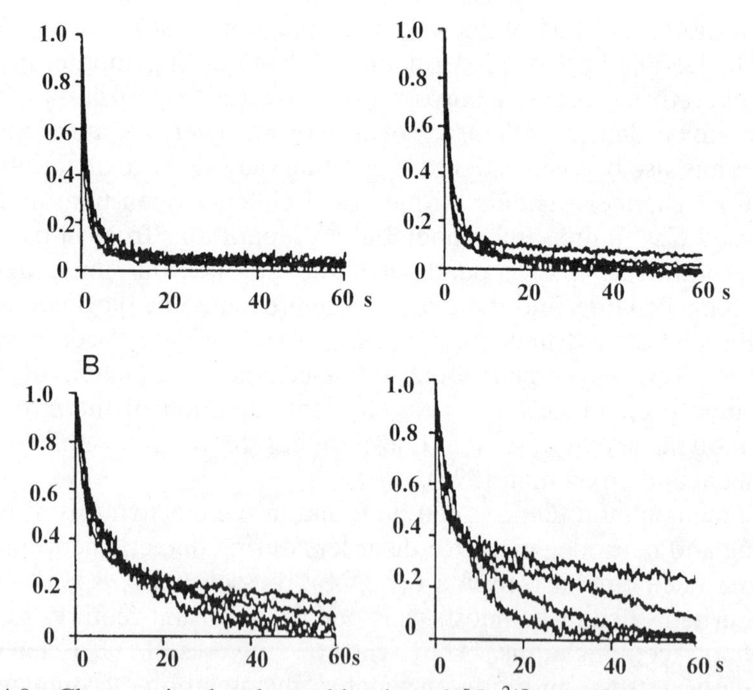

FIG 4.8 Changes in the decay kinetics of $[Ca^{2+}]_i$ transients evoked by membrane depolarization in large (A) and small (nociceptive) mice DRG neurons isolated from a control animal (*left*) and an animal with streptozotocin-induced diabetes (*right*). In each panel the responses to four depolarizations of different duration normalized to maximal current amplitude are superimposed (from Shmigol and Kostyuk, E. 1995).

Such changes may well be one of the reasons for altered nociception during diabetic neuropathy, as one of the most common complications of diabetes mellitus. In favour of the suggested mechanism of diabetic alterations in Ca^{2+} signalling are the results of experiments with long-term administration of Ca^{2+} channels blockers and insulin to the animals with experimentally induced diabetes. While subcutaneous insulin injections tended to normalize the parameters of Ca^{2+} signals modified by diabetes, L-type Ca^{2+} channels antagonists (nimodipine) did not restore their normal kinetics; on the contrary, Ca^{2+} signals induced by membrane depolarization became *increased* in peak amplitude, and often spontaneous Ca^{2+} spikes appeared in sensory neurons (Kostyuk, E. and Shmigol 1995*b*). Obviously. the extreme prolongation of $[Ca^{2+}]_i$ transients occurring as a complication of insulin-dependent diabetes is not connected to changes in the functioning of VOCC and depends mainly on alterations of enzymatic mechanisms participating in Ca^{2+} homeostasis. The nature of the steady increase in the amplitude of depolarization-induced Ca^{2+} transients as a result of chronic administration of L-type Ca^{2+} channel blockers is still an unresolved question. This increase suggests a corresponding increase in Ca^{2+} channel density, probably caused by increased expression of these channels by the cell genetic apparatus. This may be a kind of compensatory mechanism triggered by chronically decreased level of cytosolic Ca^{2+}.

CONCLUSIONS

Structural and functional changes in neuronal elements during aging can be considered as a form of negative plasticity, diminishing the effectiveness of neuronal networks to accomplish their complicated activities. Most experimental data indicate that aging is paralleled by an increase in the basal level of intracellular Ca^{2+}; in this case such elevation seems not to support neuronal survival as it occurs at early developmental stages, but to make neurons more susceptible to other pathogenic influences, like anoxia or neurodegenerative diseases. At the same time, substantial changes occur in the characteristics of Ca^{2+} signals triggered by activation of voltage- and ligand-gated ionic channels, especially in delaying the recovery of $[Ca^{2+}]_i$ to the resting level due to depression of the activity of responsible cellular systems (plasmalemmal and endoplasmic

Ca^{2+} pumps, Ca^{2+} uptake by mitochondria). Such prolongation accentuates the deleterious effects of Ca^{2+} overload and stimulates neuronal degeneration; at the same time it hinders normal information processing via surviving cells and all the integrative functions of the brain based on such processing.

5

Glia and neuronal plasticity

GENERAL FEATURES

Glial elements are the intimate partners of nerve cells during the whole life cycle, starting from the formation of neuronal networks and finishing with their aging and death. Therefore glial cells are deeply involved in all structural and functional changes which might be denoted as the plasticity of the nervous system, although their role may be very different at different stages of the life span. During neurogenesis glial elements play a leading role in directing the migration of neuronal precursors, targeting the growth of neurites, formation of nerve fibre bundles, and the establishment of synaptic connections. At the mature stage they participate in interneuronal connections, modifying the time course and amplitude of chemical signals in the synaptic clefts, liberating or accepting such signals by themselves, and even transmitting them over a distance through their own syncitial network formed by tight-junction-coupled cells. At the end of life they may be involved in neurotoxicity and neurodegeneration, probably delaying their incidence.

GLIAL ELEMENTS IN THE FORMATION OF NERVOUS SYSTEM

The leading role of glial elements in the formation of neuronal networks has been already mentioned at the beginning of the book; this role has been also extensively discussed in several reviews. Neuronal precursor cell migration and subsequent neurite outgrowth along astrocyte processes is a well documented process in the central nervous system; Schwann cells play a similar guiding and supportive role in the periphery. The interaction of adhesion molecules promotes the mobility of growth cones along glial cell surfaces, providing them with directional cues. The oligodendrocytes responsible for myelinization of neuronal processes also show complex behaviour.

An impressive finding of recent years is the fact that glial cells possess an elaborated system of voltage- and ligand-operated ion channels (see for reviews Barres *et al.* 1990; Ritchie 1992; Sontheimer 1994; Kostyuk and Verkhratsky 1995). The functional role of this system still is not quite obvious, and this has led to many speculations about its possible participation in modulation of the development and functioning of neuronal elements, taking into account that glial cells form about 90 per cent of the total cell-content of the brain.

The situation became even more intriguing after the discovery of developmental changes in the electrical and chemical sensitivity of the glial cells, most obvious in oligodendrocytes which can be easily differentiated into precursors, immature, and mature myelin-producing cells, by immunological markcrs. As was shown by Blankenfeld *et al.* (1992) and Kettenmann *et al.* (1994) on culture systems highly enriched with cells of the mouse cortical oligodendrocyte lineage, their development is marked by substantial changes in the expression of different types of VOCCs. Two different components could be distinguished in oligodendrocyte precursors identified by stage-specific monoclonal antibodies—one with activation threshold in the region of –40 mV and maximum peak at –15 mV, and another with activation threshold at –10 mV and peak at +15 mV. Fifty three per cent of the precursor cells demonstrated only the Ca^{2+} current activated at low voltages. In contrast, in mature oligodendrocytes Ca^{2+} currents always exhibited two peaks, the high-voltage one being predominant. The corresponding channels in mature cells demonstrated a very uneven distribution at the cell surface. In precursor cells membrane depolarization induced a $[Ca^{2+}]_i$ increase mainly in cellular processes, and to evoke such increase in the soma much stronger depolarization was needed. The $[Ca^{2+}]_i$ transient in the processes could be suppressed by application of 50 μM Ni^{2+}, confirming the participation of LVA Ca^{2+} channels in its generation. The somatic response was more sensitive to nifedipine (10 μM), indicating that in the somatic membrane HVA (L-type) channels could be involved in this activity. In mature cells the depolarization-induced $[Ca^{2+}]_i$ changes in the process declined and became insensitive to Ni^{2+}, indicating the developmental switch from expression of both LVA and HVA Ca^{2+} channels to entirely HVA ones (Kirischuk *et al.* 1995*b*). Figure 5.1 illustrates these changes in calcium signalling triggered by VOCC in developing mice oligodendrocytes. Prominent $[Ca^{2+}]_i$ transients triggered by low depolarizations are typical of oligodendrocyte precursor processes, being absent in soma (A); they decline in amplitude with maturation (B) being replaced by transients evoked only by strong depolarizations.

The existence of both LVA and HVA Ca^{2+} channels has also been demonstrated in Schwann cells from the organotypic culture of mice dorsal root ganglia (Amadee *et al.* 1991). Here the situation became

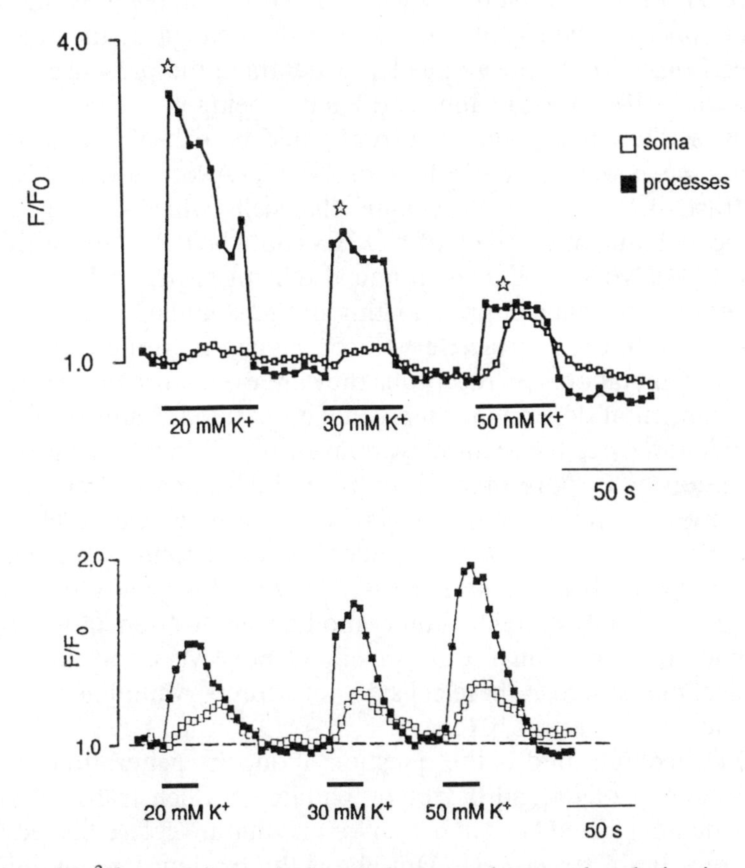

FIG 5.1 $[Ca^{2+}]_i$ transients induced by membrane depolarizations in oligodendrocyte precursor (A) and mature (B) cells. The transients were evoked by application of external solutions containing different concentrations of KCl and measured in processes and soma by fura-2 emission; changes in $[Ca^{2+}]_i$ level are expressed as the relationship between light emission at 360 and 380 nm (Kirischuk 1996).

complicated by the fact that expression of Ca^{2+} channels was recorded only if nerve cells also were present in the culture, indicating the presence of some unidentified messengers between developing neuronal and glial elements.

A complicated developmental and cell-specific programme of the expression of VOCCs has been revealed in astrocytes. Again LVA and dihydropyridine-sensitive HVA Ca^{2+} currents were demonstrated in these cells in culture, their expression being dependent on some outside messengers including those generated by co-cultured neurons (Barres *et al.* 1989; Corvalan *et al.* 1990). Attempts to record these currents *in situ* were unsuccessful. However, recently measurements on identified glial cells (obviously astrocytes) in thin brain slices from mice hippocampus have identified the presence of both LVA and HVA Ca^{2+} channels, the latter being probably of several types, as the corresponding current could be partially inhibited by nifedipine as well as by ω-conotoxin GVIA (Akopian *et al.* 1996). In contrast, in cerebellar Bergmann glial cells which belong to the astrocyte family no activity of VOCCs could be detected (Kirischuk *et al.* 1994). No VOCCs were found also in microglial cells.

Another mechanism participating in the stimulation of glial cells and generation of intracellular Ca^{2+} signals is formed by ligand-operated metabotropic receptors; they are even more numerous and developmental-dependent than voltage-operated channels. Thus, in oligodendrocytes transient elevations of $[Ca^{2+}]_i$ can be triggered by activation of P_2 purinoreceptors by ATP, leading to liberation of Ca^{2+} from intracellular stores via $InsP_3$-sensitive release channels. This mechanism could be revealed only in late precursor and mature cells, not in early precursors (Kirischuk *et al.* 1995*c*), as illustrated in Fig. 5.2. Neither caffeine nor ryanodine application induced any changes in intracellular Ca^{2+} in oligodendrocytes, indicating that intracellular stores in these cells do not express ryanodine receptors and cannot generate CICR.

Quite complicated is the question about the generation of Ca^{2+} transients in oligodendrocytes by glutamate. Such transients have been demonstrated both in precursor and mature cells cultured from different brain structures. Data about the existence of mGluRs in glial cells are very limited. Therefore it is suggested that they can be triggered by membrane depolarization due to activation of AMPA/kainate ionotropic receptors and subsequent Ca^{2+} influx through VOCCs (Borges *et al.* 1994); on the other hand there are indications that AMPA/kainate receptors in glial cells can have, by themselves,

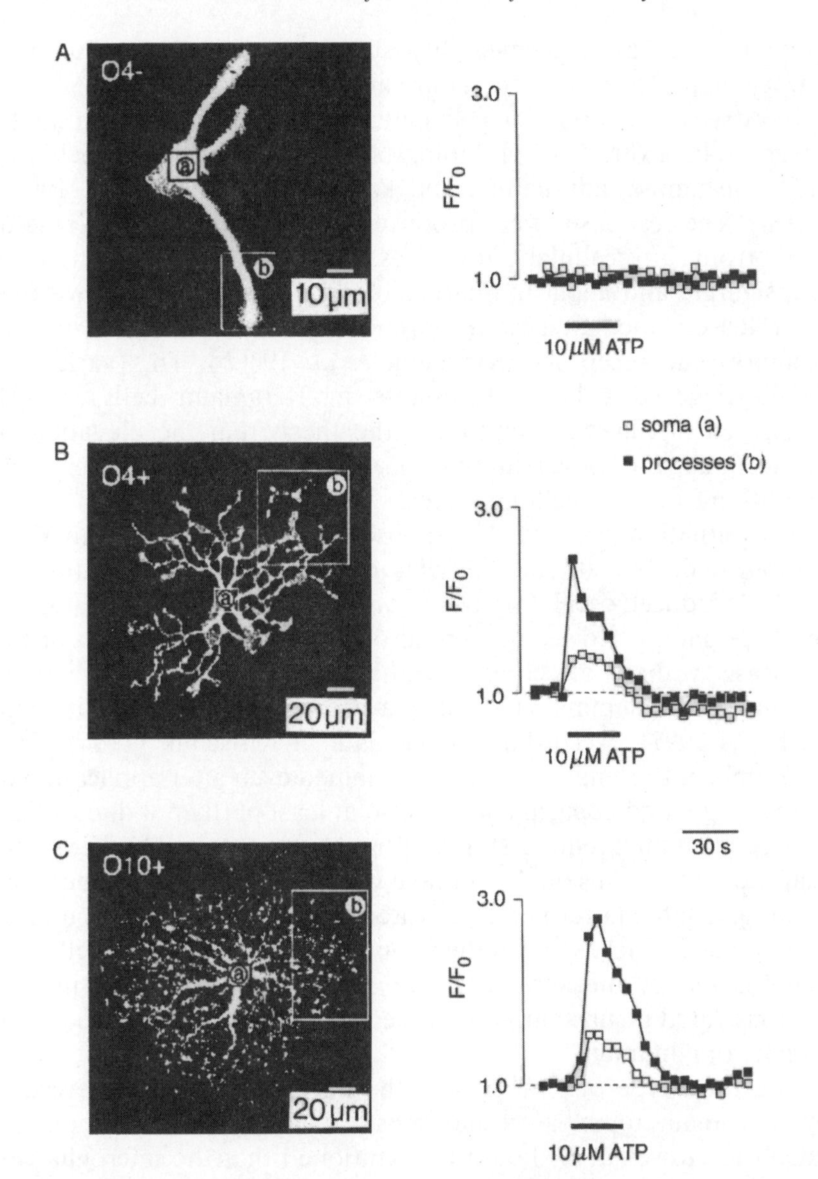

FIG 5.2 $[Ca^{2+}]_i$ transients induced in oligodendrocyte precursors (A, B) and mature (C) cells by the application of ATP, triggering Ca^{2+} release from intracellular stores. The figure is constructed in the same way as Fig. 5.1. Images of the corresponding cells (the developmental stage of which has been identified by antibodies of the O-series) are shown on the left (Kirischuk 1996).

quite high calcium permeability sufficient to induce substantial intracellular Ca^{2+} transients (Holzwarth *et al.* 1994).

In astrocytes (Bergmann cells) intracellular Ca^{2+} transients can be triggered by a variety of physiologically-active substances, including ATP, histamine, adrenaline, and kainate (Kirischuk *et al.* 1995*a*, 1996*a*). The responses were produced by $InsP_3$-mediated release of Ca^{2+} from intracellular stores, as they could be inhibited by thapsigargin and heparin; pharmacological analysis has shown that the release is mediated via α_1-adreno, H_1-histamine, and P_2-purino metabotropic receptors (Kirischuk *et al.* 1966*b*). This variety of ligand-triggered calcium transients in Bergmann cells is well illustrated in Fig. 5.3, confirming the thesis that the elevation of intracellular Ca^{2+} level in this case is almost entirely due to its liberation from intracellular stores.

The situation with glial responses to glutamate is somewhat complicated. In rat cortical glial cells in culture, activation of mGluRs induced oscillatory elevations of $[Ca^{2+}]_i$ which were blocked by thapsigargin. However, Cd^{2+} also suppressed the plateau of the response, without affecting its initial rise. Thus some Ca^{2+} influx through plasmalemmal channels may be also involved (Mathie and Richards 1997). According to the data of Kirischuk (1966), Ca^{2+} transients in Bergmann glial cells remained even after application of thapsigargin and heparin and are also at least partly not due to Ca^{2+} release from intracellular stores. It has been suggested by Kirischuk that the mechanisms of Ca^{2+} uptake via the Na^+/Ca^{2+} exchanger may be involved, the latter being activated by sodium-dependent uptake of glutamate which is one of the important functions of glial cells (see below). Direct measurements on Bergmann cells have in fact demonstrated a substantial increase of $[Na^+]_i$ during application of kainate or glutamate.

The third type of glial tissue—the microglia—is less interesting for our main topic, as it has mostly a defensive (macrophage) function. However, it should be mentioned that the microglia can also express metabotropic P_2-receptors and generate intracellular Ca^{2+} transients, which probably trigger their transformation into macrophages. The only other factor which can generate such transients is the complement-factor C5a. The liberation of Ca^{2+} ions comes from $InsP_3$-sensitive stores and may be amplified by additional activation of Ca-release-activated (CRAC) channels in their plasmalemma.

Although the exact types of VOCC and ligand-operated channels

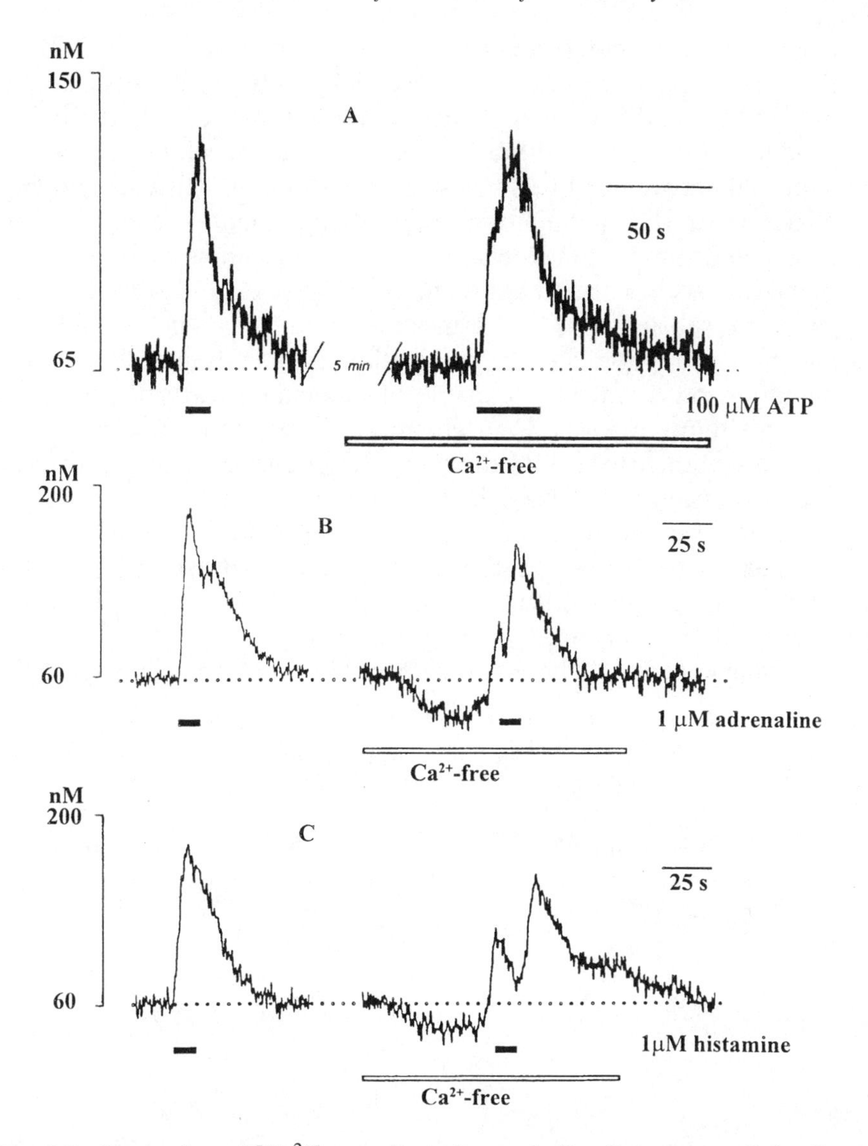

FIG 5.3 Examples of $[Ca^{2+}]_i$ transients in cerebellar Bergmann glial cells evoked by external applications of 100 μM ATP (A), 1 μM adrenaline (B) and 1 μM histamine (C). Application time is indicated by black bars. Left columns show transients under control conditions, and right columns after 2 min slice superfusion with Ca^{2+} free solution, shown by open bars (from Kirischuk *et al.* 1994).

in glial cells have not yet been exactly determined and the data about their expression are often controversial (probably because of the extreme variability of glial elements), the specific role of Ca^{2+} influx produced by them at different stages of the development of the neuronal network can be suggested. The simultaneously developing oligodendrocytes definitely change their function, as might be expected from dramatic changes in the mechanisms of calcium signalling. As has been mentioned, the mature oligodendrocytes can generate substantial Ca^{2+} transients in their soma, capable of inducing retraction and fragmentation of membrane sheets; the immature ones are more capable of inducing growth of processes by activation of LVA Ca^{2+} channels in response to even small depolarizations (local elevations of $[K^+]_o$) and generation of local $[Ca^{2+}]_i$ transients, thus participating in some way in the development of neuronal connections (cf. Benjamins and Nedelkoska 1996).

Figure 5.4 summarizes the existing data about developmental changes in the mechanisms of intracellular signalling in cells of the oligodendrocyte lineage.

Similar functional changes may occur in Schwann cells, especially

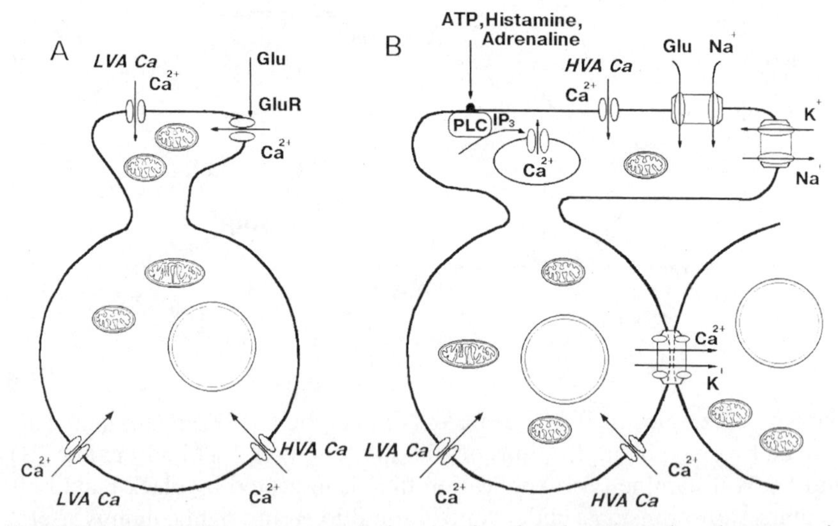

FIG 5.4 Schematic representation of developmental changes in intracellular signalling in cells of oligodendrocytic lineage. A–progenitor cell, B–mature cell. *LVA Ca and HVA Ca*–corresponding voltage-operated Ca^{2+} channels, *GluR*–ionotropic glutamate channels, *PLC*–phospholypase C, *GLU, N*–sodium glutamate cotransporter, K^+, Na^+–Na^+/K^+ exchanger, *Ca^{2+}, K^+–gap junction.*

in their perisynaptic elements which cover the neuromuscular junctions and which change their activity substantially during innervation and denervation. Schwann cells are known to be capable of producing and releasing neuromodulators, this process being modulated by changes in gene expression in these cells triggered by alterations in cAMP or $[Ca^{2+}]_i$ levels. Such release may an important factor in synapse formation, maturation, and maintenance (cf. Giulian 1993; Vernadakis 1996).

GLIA–NEURONAL INTERACTIONS AND SYNAPTIC PLASTICITY

In the mature neuronal network the main role of glial elements in neuronal activity can be executed by astrocytic processes which often closely approach the synaptic junctions and even sometimes embrace the whole neuron, as in the case of Bergmann glial cells and Purkinje neurons in the cerebellum or Muller cells in the retina.

Initially the role of glial elements in synaptic transmission was suggested to be a mechanism for stabilizing the ionic environment in the synaptic space by removing excessive accumulation of ions and transmitters occurring during neuronal activity and preventing possible alterations in synaptic processes. For instance, it has been shown by direct measurements that K^+ ions can accumulate in substantial amounts in the extracellular space during neuronal activity, sufficient to depolarize the neuronal elements. Reduction of K^+ uptake in glia by extracellular Cs^+ has been shown to cause epileptiform activity in hippocampal structures and prevent the maintenance of long-term depression (Janigro *et al.* 1997). In fact, effective accumulation of K^+ by astrocytic processes has been recorded in astrocytes (Hertz 1978) and retinal Muller cells (Newman *et al.* 1984). Strong electric coupling between astrocytes, in contrast with much weaker coupling between oligodendrocytes (cf. Kettenmann and Ransom 1988) would make a syncythium from astrocytes facilitating rapid transport of K^+ away from areas of their focal extracellular accumulation.

Later substantial differences in this respect were found between different brain structures. There are subpopulations of astrocytes with different coupling possibilities; the latter was found to be weakest in spinal cord, higher in brain stem and cortex, and highest in the optic nerve (Lee *et al.* 1994). This may reflect their functional heterogeneity in respect of supporting ionic equilibrium in the extraneuronal space. Cell coupling may play a role in increasing extracellular ionic buffering, while uncoupled cells may function in a more focal manner (see below).

The regulation of the extracellular Ca^{2+} level may be a related function of astroglia. As has been already stated, glutamate and other neurotransmitters can trigger substantial $[Ca^{2+}]_i$ transients and oscillations in astrocytes; due to gap-junctions they can form propagated Ca^{2+} waves. As VOCCs are also present in astrocytes, they can form an additional mechanism for influx of Ca^{2+} from the extracellular space. Due to the presence of gap junctions, intracellular Ca^{2+} waves may propagate both within astrocytes, occurring in cell bodies and processes, as well as between individual astrocytes (Dani *et al.* 1992; Porter and McCarthy 1995). The participation of phospholipase C, $InsP_3$ production and involvement of internal calcium stores are also important for the generation of calcium waves in astrocytes (Venance *et al.* 1997). In retinal glial cells such waves have been studied in detail. It has been shown that they propagate at a velocity of 23 $\mu m\ s^{-1}$, persist in the absence of extracellular Ca^{2+} but are largely abolished by thapsigargin and intracellular heparin indicating that Ca^{2+} release from intracellular stores is important for their support; they can travel synchronously in astrocytes and Müller cells suggesting a functional leakage between these two types of glial cell (Newman and Zahs 1997).

Finally, at glutamatergic synapses glutamate can also be effectively taken up by astrocytes, terminating its trans-synaptic action. Glutamate is co-transported with Na^+ and metabolized to glutamine by glutamine synthetase which is predominantly localized in glial cells (Norenberg and Martinez-Serrano 1979). The uptake of glutamate is followed by a chain of subsequent enzymatic reactions. The parallel increase in intracellular Na^+ activates Na^+/K^+ ATPase and glycolysis, resulting in increased lactate production in astrocytes. The latter can be released back into the extracellular space and taken up by neuronal elements, probably serving as an additional energy substrate. This mechanism can be an important component preventing, to a certain extent, the overproduction of glutamate and its toxicity during ischaemia; at the same time it can change its function in the opposite direction when the glial cells became overloaded with glutamate and the Na^+-dependent uptake reverses into its release. Transport of glutamate into astrocytes can also be inhibited by arachidonic acid synthesized in them under the activation of the above mentioned metabotropic glutamate and purinergic receptors (Glowinski *et al.* 1994).

The possibility of inhibition or reversal of the uptake processes in astrocytes definitely indicates that not only do they play a defensive role in the functioning of synaptic connections preventing them from being overloaded by intermediates, but they also play a more active role by releasing synaptic transmitters and modulators and inducing in this way plastic changes in synaptic activity. The induction of Ca^{2+} signals in astrocytes or their processes can lead to glutamate release from them; this phenomenon may be of a propagated nature if a wave of Ca^{2+} increase starts to propagate from astrocyte to astrocyte and affect neurons adjacent to them. Consequently synaptic efficacy will increase as the perisynaptic concentration of glutamate rises. Such a facilitatory effect may be modulated by other neurotransmitters which trigger via metabotropic receptors the activation of phospholipase A_2 that liberates arachidonic acid, inhibiting glutamate re-uptake. Release of K^+ ions into the perisynaptic space which can occur during the generation of Ca^{2+} transients in astrocytes via K^+ efflux from them through the opening of Ca^{2+}-activated K^+ channels may exert up to a point an additional facilitatory effect by depolarizing the corresponding neuronal structures. Excessive accumulation of $[K^+]_o$ will again reverse the facilitatory effect into depression (cf. review by Finkbeiner 1993).

The close functional interrelation between astrocytes and neurons is especially demonstrative in the case of cerebellar Purkinje neurons and Bergmann glial cells, which in fact embrace each other by their processes and express almost similar examples of $[Ca^{2+}]_i$ transients triggered by metabotropic receptors. Obviously, in this case any type of chemical synaptic activity will activate responses in both structures with vast possibilities of mutual interaction. This close parallelism in the activity of a neuronal and glial structure is well illustrated in Fig. 5.5.

Astrocytes may play a different role in neuronal functioning in the aging brain. It is known that proliferation of astrocytes occurs in some areas of the aging brain; however the question whether such proliferation is a consequence of neuronal death or a compensatory phenomenon preventing death is still open. In any case, recent investigations have shown that cell cultures derived from aged brains can stimulate various stages of astrocyte differentiation *in vivo*, indicating that glial cells can express progenitor properties through-

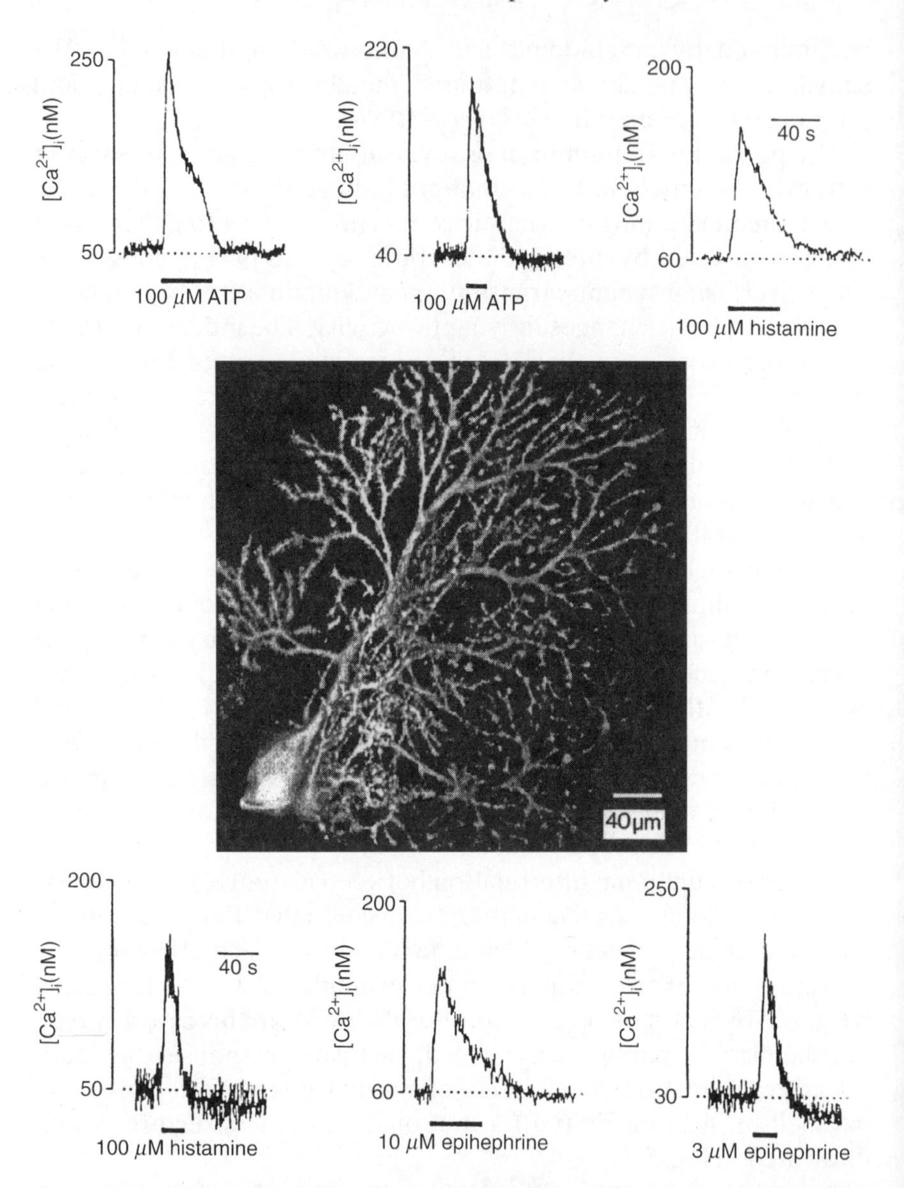

FIG 5.5 Expression of identical metabotropic receptors in a cerebellar Purkinje neuron (*left*) and adjacent Bergmann glial cell (*right*). $[Ca^{2+}]_i$ transients were evoked by external application of 100 μM ATP, 100 μM histamine, and 3 μM epinephrine. An image of both cells stained with Lucifer yellow is presented in the centre (Kirischuk 1996).

out their whole life span and respond actively even at their final stages (Vernadakis and Kentroti 1994).

CONCLUSIONS

Glial cells are intimate partners of neurons throughout the life span of the nervous system and are deeply involved in plastic changes of the functioning of neuronal elements. The properties of all types of glial element by themselves undergo substantial developmental changes. Thus, in developing oligodendrocytes principal changes in the spectrum of expressed ionic channels occur during maturation, enabling them to fulfil their multiple role in guiding neurite outgrowth, establishment of synaptic contacts, and myelinization of nerve fibres. The astrocytes are more involved in prolonged changes in the functioning of mature neuronal connections. On one hand, they can effectively stabilize the composition of the perisynaptic space by absorbing extracellular K^+ and Ca^{2+} ions as well as transmitters (glutamate) and equilibrating them across the astrocytic net via a flexible system of gap junctions, thus protecting neurons from over-excitation and excitotoxicity. On the other, they can produce Ca^{2+}-triggered liberation of glutamate which to a certain point will enhance synaptic efficacy. However, this potentiating effect may turn into a depressing one if it becomes the major route of excessive non-synaptic glutamate release, finally leading to neuronal death, as happens in hypoxic–ischaemic conditions.

6

Common features in the mechanisms of different forms of neuronal plasticity

The data presented in the preceding chapters demonstrate that persistent changes in the functional properties of neuronal elements (neuronal plasticity) are a general feature of the functioning of the nervous system. The expression of such changes is highly dependent on the developmental stage of the organisms—they are more drastic and generalized during formation of the neuronal network, more localized and specialized in its mature state, and again become generalized in the decaying phase of the life cycle. Some reversal to initial features of plasticity is possible after brain damage and incidence of regenerative processes, provided that enough neuronal elements survived and retained the capability of regeneration.

Despite this multiplicity in the expression of plastic changes in neuronal functioning, the cellular mechanisms which trigger or regulate complex changes in neuronal structure and action include common basic steps, the most general of which are temporal elevations of the intracellular level of Ca^{2+} ions (calcium 'transients' or 'signals'). The most striking feature of this role of calcium signalling, despite its extremely generalized character, is its capability to affect extremely specialized cellular processes and exert on them both up- and down-regulatory effects. The possibility of such specificity of action on target as well as in time and sign are provided by several features of the intracellular calcium-signalling machinery.

SPATIAL ARRANGEMENTS OF CALCIUM SIGNALLING IN THE CELL

Despite the small size of nerve cells and the possibilities of free diffusion of Ca^{2+} in the cytosol, substantial intracellular spatial and temporal Ca^{2+} gradients may still appear during cellular activity. The formation of such local patches may be promoted by the existence of spatial limitations for free diffusion, like dendritic spines in which the possibility of the generation of localized high-amplitude Ca^{2+} transients has been directly shown (Holmes 1990; Muller and Connor 1991; Connor *et al.* 1994; Eilers *et al.* 1996). According to Denk *et al.* (1995), individual spines are capable of independent calcium activation; moreover, two distinct spine populations could be distinguished by their opposite responses to membrane potential changes. Similar possibilities are present also in fine dendritic arborizations.

Another way of increasing the effectiveness of the action of Ca^{2+} transients is close apposition of Ca channels and target structures. An example of highest effectiveness is the direct coupling between sarcolemmal L-type Ca channels and Ca^{2+}-release channels (ryanodine receptors) in the sarcoplasmic reticulum of striated muscle fibre; in this case the displacement of the gating charges in the former leads to Ca^{2+} release, without the necessity to inject these ions through the plasmalemma. Recently the possibility of such direct coupling has been suggested for some neuronal structures, for example crayfish abdominal ganglion neurons (Brown 1996) and mouse cerebellar Purkinje cells (Shimahara *et al.* 1996). However, at least in mammalian sensory neurons careful testing could not reveal any indications of direct coupling, and influx of Ca^{2+} through plasmalemmal channels was always the prerequisite of the induction of CICR (Kostyuk and Shmigol 1997). An oppositely directed interaction mechanism between ryanodine receptors and VOCCs has been recently suggested for cerebellar granule neurons: activation of mGluR1 receptors here induced a large, oscillating increase in the L-type Ba^{2+} current which could be mimicked by caffeine and blocked by ryanodine; it was independent of $InsP_3$ and classical protein kinases and was not triggered by the CICR mechanism, as it persisted even in inside-out membrane patches (Chavis *et al.* 1996).

An impressive example of the effectiveness of spatial apposition has recently been obtained on adrenal aldosterone-secreting cells, in which Ca^{2+} influx through T-type Ca channels occurs in such close proximity to mitochondria that it evokes selective increase in intramitochondrial Ca^{2+} level necessary for stimulation of steroidgenesis (Rossier *et al.* 1996). A more general example of spatial apposition is the co-localization of Ca^{2+} channels and release sites in synaptic terminals and neuroendocrine cells. Such co-localization may lead to substantial local elevations (up to micromolar levels) of $[Ca^{2+}]_i$ necessary for triggering the low-affinity Ca^{2+}-dependent processes involved in exocytosis (cf. Llinas *et al.* 1992; Chow *et al.* 1994; Klingauf and Neher 1997).

Activation of Ca^{2+}-release mechanisms can be an additional factor in local amplification of calcium signals, especially if the Ca^{2+} stores are located close to the sites of Ca^{2+} entry. For instance, such local Ca^{2+} release from subsurface cisternae triggered by $InsP_3$ has been recently demonstrated in pituitary gonadotrophs, raising $[Ca^{2+}]_i$ near the exocytotic site 5-fold above cell average (Tse *et al.* 1997). Substantial prolongation of calcium signals by Ca^{2+} release can be also an important factor in stressing their functional importance, as it has been demonstrated on CA3 hippocampal pyramidal neurons (Miller *et al.* 1996). It should be specially indicated that the participation of such amplification mechanisms is highly specialized for certain types of neuronal structure. Thus, $InsP_3$-triggered Ca^{2+} release activated by extracellular ATP, presumably via metabotropic P_{2Y} receptors, is highly expressed in large DRG neurons in the mouse (Svichar *et al.* 1997*a*) but completely absent from small ones transmitting predominantly nociceptive signals (Svichar *et al.* 1997*b*). In Purkinje neurons the endoplasmic reticulum subcompartments themselves demonstrate highly heterogeneous distribution of $InsP_3$ receptors and Ca^{2+}–ATPase (Takei *et al.* 1992).

Localized changes in the effectiveness of calcium signalling can also be induced by an opposite arrangement—co-localization of sources of Ca^{2+} influx and enzymatic mechanisms which prevent excessive Ca^{2+} elevation in the cytosol either by extruding ions back into extracellular space or down-regulating the activity of VOCCs. Such self-association of the PMCA-pump has been shown in special parts of the total plasma membrane, in close association with VOCCs (cf. Monteith and Roufogalis 1995; Hillman *et al.* 1996); another example is the co-localization of VOCCs and phosphatase 2B (calcineurine) which effectively down-regulates L- and N-type channels in different neuronal cells (Lukyanetz *et al.* 1996; Lukyanetz 1997).

Finally, a most sophisticated example of functional co-localization of sources and targets of Ca^{2+} ions has been recently suggested for exocytosis—it has been shown that the secretory granules themselves have the properties of Ca^{2+} stores (Gerasimenko *et al.* 1996*a*) and can release Ca^{2+} into the cytosol via a messenger-mediated pathway following agonist binding; such release might be quite important for the amplification of localized cytosolic calcium signals which initiate exocytosis (cf. reviews by Petersen 1996*a*, *b*).

SPECIFIC BINDING TO DIFFERENT MOLECULAR STRUCTURES AND DIFFERENT SITES IN THE SAME STRUCTURE

Another way to promote specific action of Ca^{2+} on certain cellular mechanisms is based on differences in the affinity of the Ca^{2+}-dependent enzymatic systems involved. A highly illustrative example of such specificity has been obtained in our already mentioned investigations of the down-regulation of the activity of HVA Ca^{2+} channels by changes in the basal level of $[Ca^{2+}]_i$. Ca^{2+}-buffered solutions with different levels of free Ca^{2+} were used for perfusion of identified snail neuron, enabling estimation of the concentration-dependence of the down-regulatory effect of intracellular Ca^{2+} on calcium currents previously potentiated by activation of the cAMP–PKA enzymatic chain. This dependence clearly followed a biphasic curve representing two Langmuir's isotherms with different dissociation constants ($K_{d1} = 0.063$ μM and $K_{d2} = 1$ μM) manifesting Ca^{2+}-dependent activation of two enzymatic reactions involved in the modulation of channel functioning. For separation and quantitative evaluation of the participation of different enzymes in these effects, a similar approach was used in the presence of specific enzyme antagonists. It proved that the corresponding reactions represent activation of Ca^{2+}-dependent form of phosphodiesterase (PhDE) and Ca^{2+}-dependent phosphatase (calcineurin). The natural course of events may be summarized in the following way: at resting conditions ($[Ca^{2+}]_i$ below 0.1 μM) Ca^{2+} channels can be effectively up-regulated by cAMP–PKA-dependent phosphorylation. However, if $[Ca^{2+}]_i$ rises, first PhDE becomes activated, preventing further up-regulation of channels. If $[Ca^{2+}]_i$ nevertheless continues to rise and reaches micromolar levels, effective channel dephosphorylation by calcineurin is added which finally may bring them to complete silence (cf. Kostyuk and Lukyanetz 1993, 1994).

Another example is Ca^{2+} accumulation and mobilization by different intracellular stores (mitochondrial and microsomal). Maximal Ca^{2+} accumulation in mitochondria is higher than in the endoplasmic reticulum; however, it starts only when $[Ca^{2+}]_i$ approaches a quite high level (≈0.5 μM), leading to substantial slow-down of both rise and recovery of calcium transients if they reach such high amplitude and changing the degree of activation of Ca^{2+}-dependent intracellular processes (data of Friel and Tsien 1994, on sympathetic neurons). Various Ca^{2+} mediators can preferentially release Ca^{2+}

only from one of these stores, also inducing substantial modifications of the calcium transients (observations of Huang and Chueh 1996 on rat cerebellum). Differences in spatial distribution of mitochondrial and non-mitochondrial stores, quite prominent between neuronal somata, growth cones or synaptic terminals, and dendritic arborizations may also influence to a large extent the shape of evoked calcium transients. This has been well illustrated on cerebellar Purkinje neurons (Kano *et al.* 1995; Eilers *et al.* 1995).

The structural variability of HVA Ca^{2+} channels and the presence of substantial differences in their sensitivity to modulatory factors may also serve as a mechanism responsible for selective effects, taking into account differential distribution of various channel types in neuronal structures. For instance, some factors define clustering of L-type Ca^{2+} channels at the branching points of dendrites and N-type channels at the active zones of the synapses in hippocampal pyramidal cells (Westenbroek *et al.* 1992); such spatial patterns, existing also in other types of cells, induce specific patterns of $[Ca^{2+}]_i$ increase in these structures caused by activation of VOCCs (cf. Bischofberger and Schild 1995).

Definitely, combinations of all the above mentioned factors can not only modify a wide range of the spatial and temporal characteristics of calcium signals, but induce opposite effects. In some cases Ca^{2+} ions exert on the corresponding substrate a clear bell-shaped concentration-dependent effect, for instance, on the mechanism of $InsP_3$-induced Ca^{2+} release (Bezprozvanny *et al.* 1991). This transformation from facilitation to depression opens even wider possibilities for changing the functional role of calcium signals, depending on combinations of various types of activity going on in the cell.

INVOLVEMENT OF GENETIC MECHANISMS AND ACTIVATION (OR INHIBITION) OF SYNTHESIS OF NEW PROTEINS

Most fundamental changes in the functional properties of neuronal elements are connected with alterations in the expression of ion channels, receptors, and intracellular messenger systems. The mechanisms inducing such alterations are still described mainly in general terms as triggered by activation (or suppression) of gene expression, involving the system of immediate–early genes (IEGs).

Intracellular Ca^{2+} transients again seem to be an important element in these events, and it is now becoming evident that their participation may be mediated not only by intermediate cytoplasmic substrates which later became translocated into the nucleus (like MAP kinases), but also by direct intervention in nuclear processes. As has been already mentioned in Chapter 3, the nuclear envelop by itself forms a calcium store which can accumulate Ca^{2+} ions due to activity of Ca^{2+}ATPase present in its outer membrane and release them into the nucleoplasm due to activation of cyclic ADP–ribose- and $InsP_3$-sensitive channels specifically localized in the inner membrane (Gerasimenko *et al.* 1995, 1996*b*). Of course, further work must be directed towards establishing the exact function of these Ca^{2+} signals. The cell nucleus has even been described as an 'Eldorado for future calcium research', especially for studies of calmodulin and other Ca^{2+}-dependent enzymes as specific intranuclear modulation targets (Santella 1996). A promising approach is a recent detailed analysis of $InsP_3$ receptors in the nuclear envelope, including their single-channel kinetics, inactivation, and spatial distribution (Mak and Foskett 1997).

References

Adams, B. A. and Beam, K. G. (1989). A novel calcium current in dysgenic skeletal muscle. *J. Gen. Physiol.*, **94**, 429–44.

Akaike, N., Kostyuk, P. G., and Osipchuk, Y. V. (1989). Dihiydropyridine-sensitive low-threshold calcium channels in isolated rat hypothalamic neurones. *J. Physiol. (London)*, **412**, 181–95.

Akita, T., Loyner, R. W., Lu, C., Kumar, R., and Yartzell, H. C. (1994). Developmental changes in modulation of calcium currents of rabbit ventricular cells by phosphodiesterase inhibitors. *Circulation,* **90**, 469–78.

Akopian, A., Kressin, K., Derouiche, A. and Steinhauser, C. (1996). Identified glial cells in the early postnatal mouse hippocampus display different types of CA^{++} currents. *Glia*, **17**, 181–94.

Al-Mohanna, F. A., Cave, J., and Bolsover, S. R. (1992). A narrow window of intracellular calcium concentration is optimal for neurite outgrowth in rat sensory neurones. *Develop. Brain Res.*, **70**, 287–90.

Amato, A., Al-Mohanna, F. A., and Bolsover, S. R. (1996). Spatial organization of calcium dynamics in growth cones of sensory neurones. *Develop. Brain Res.*, **92**, 101–10.

Amadee, T., Ellie, E., Dupouy, B., and Vincent, J. D. (1991). Voltage-dependent calcium and potassium channels in Schwann cells cultured from dorsal root ganglia of the mouse. *J. Physiol. (London),* **441**, 35–56.

An, R. H., Davies, M. P., Doevendans, P. A., Kubalak, S. W., Bangalore, R., Chien, K. R., *et al.* (1996). Developmental changes in β-adrenergic modulation of L-type Ca^{2+} channels in embryonic mouse heart. *Circ. Res.,* **78**, 371–8.

Arispe, N., Pollard, H. B. and Rojas, E. (1994). The ability of amyloid β-protein [AβP (1–40)] to form Ca^{++} channels provides a mechanism for neuronal death in Alzheimer's disease. *Ann. New York Acad. Sci.*, **747**, 256–66.

Artola, A. and Singer, W. (1993). Long-term depression of excitatory synaptic transmission and its relationship to long-term potentiation. *Trends Neurosci.,* **16**, 480–7.

Artola, A., Hensch, T., and Singer, W. (1996). Calcium induced long-term depression in the visual cortex of the rat in vitro. *J. Neurosci.,* **76**, 984–94.

Augustine, G. J., Betz, H., Bommert, K., Charlton, M. P., DeBello, W. M., Hans, M., *et al.* (1994). Molecular pathways for presynaptic calcium signalling. In: *Molecular and cellular mechanisms of neurotransmitters release*, (ed. L. Stjarne *et al.*), pp. 139–53. Raven, New York.

Bandtlow, C. E., Schmidt, M. F., Hassinger, T. D., Schwab, M. E., and Kater, B. (1993). Role of intracellular calcium in NI-35-evoked collapse of neuronal growth cones. *Science*, **259**, 80–3.

Bangalore, R. and Triggle, D. J. (1995). Age-dependent changes in voltage-gated calcium channels and ATP-dependent potassium channels in Fisher 344 rats. *Gen. Pharmacol.*, **26**, 1237–42.

Bargas, J., Surmeier, D. J. and Kitai, S. T. (1991). High- and low-voltage activated calcium currents are expressed by neurons cultured from embryonic rat neostriatum. *Brain Res.* **1991**, 70–4.

Barish, M. E. (1986). Differentiation of voltage-gated potassium current and modulation of excitability in cultured amphibian spinal neurones. *J. Physiol. (London)*, **375**, 229–50.

Barish, M. E. (1991). Increases in intracellular calcium ion concentration during depolarization of cultured embryonic *Xenopus* spinal neurones. *J. Physiol. (London)*, **444**, 545–65.

Barish, M. E. and Mansdorf, N. B. (1991). Development of intracellular calcium responses to depolarization and to kainate and *N*-methyl-d-aspartate in cultured mouse hippocampal neurons. *Develop. Brain Res.*, **63**, 53–61.

Barish, M. E., Mansdorf, N. B., and Raissada, S. S. (1991). γ-Interferon promotes differentiation of cultured cortical and hippocampal neurons. *Develop. Biology*, **144**, 412–23.

Barres, B. A., Chun, L. L. Y., and Corey, D. P. (1989). Calcium current in cortical astrocytes: induction by cAMP and neurotransmitters and permissive effect of serum factors. *J. Neurosci.*, **9**, 3169–75.

Barres, B. A., Chun, L. L. Y., and Corey, D. P. (1990). Ion channels in vertebrate glia. *Annu. Rev. Neurosci.*, **13**, 441–74.

Basarsky, T. A., Parpura, V., and Haydon, P. G. (1994). Hippocampal synaptogenesis in cell culture: developmental time course of synapse formation, calcium influx, and synaptic protein distribution. *J. Neurosci.*, **14**, 6402–11.

Bashir, Z. I., and Collingridge, G. L. (1992). Synaptic plasticity: long-term potentiation in the hippocampus. *Curr. Opin. Neurobiol.*, **2**, 328–35.

Baumgold, J., and Spector, I. (1987). Development of sodium channel protein during chemically induced differentiation of neuroblastoma cells. *J. Neurochem.*, **48**, 1264–9.

Bear, M. F. and Abraham, W. C. (1996). Long-term depression in hippocampus. *Annu. Rev. Neurosci.*, **19**, 437–62.

Beatty, D. M., Sands, S. A., Morris, S. J., and Chronwall, B. M. (1996). Types and activities of voltage-operated channels change during development of rat pituitary neurointermediate lobe. *Int. J. Dev. Neurosci.*, **14**, 597–612.

Benjamins, J. A. and Nedelkoska, L. (1996). Release of intracellular calcium stores leads to retraction of membrane sheets and cell death in mature mouse oligodendrocytes. *Neurochem. Res.,* **21**, 471–9.

Bezprozvanny, I., Watras, J., and Ehrlich, B. E. (1991). Bell-shaped calcium-response curves of Ins(1,4,5)P_3 and calcium-gated channels from endoplasmic reticulum of cerebellum. *Nature,* **351**, 751–4.

Bickmayer, U., Muller, E., and Wiegand, H. (1993). Development of calcium currents in cultures of mouse spinal cord and dorsal root ganglion neurones. *NeuroReport,* **4**, 131–4.

Biessels, G. and Gispen, W. H. (1996). The calcium hypothesis of brain aging and neurodegenerative disorders: significance in diabetic neuropathy. *Life Sci.,* **59**, 379–87.

Bischofberger, J. and Schild, D. (1995). Different spatial patterns of [Ca^{2+}] increase caused by N- and L-type Ca^{2+} channel activation in frog olfactory bulb neurones. *J. Physiol. (London),* **487**, 305–17.

Blair, L. A. C. and Dionne, V. E. (1985). Developmental acquisition of Ca^{2+}-sensitivity by K^+ channels in spinal neurones. *Nature,* **315**, 329–31.

Blankenfeld, G., Verkhratsky, A., and Kettenmann, H. (1992). Ca^{2+} channel expression in the oligodendrocyte lineage. *Eur. J. Neurosci.,* **4**, 1035–48.

Bliss, T. V. P. and Lomo, T. (1973). Long-lasting potentiation of synaptic transmission in the dentate area of anaesthetized rabbit following stimulation of the perforant path. *J. Physiol. (London),* **232**, 357–74.

Blond, O., Daniel, H., Otani, S., Jaillard, D., and Crepel, F. (1997). Presynaptic and postsynaptic effects of nitric oxide donors at synapses between parallel fibres and Purkinje cells: involvement in cerebellar long-term depression. *Neuroscience,* **77**, 945–54.

Bolshakov, V. Y. and Siegelbaum, S. A. (1994). Postsynaptic induction and presynaptic expression of hippocampal long-term depression. *Science,* **264**, 1148–52.

Borde, M., Cazalets, J. R., and Buno, W. (1995). Activity-dependent response depression in rat hippocampal CA1 pyramidal neurons in vitro. *J. Neurophysiol.,* **74**, 1714–29.

Borges, K. I., Ohlemeyer, C., Trotter, J., and Kettenmann, H. (1994). AMPA/kainate receptor activation in murine oligodendrocyte precursor cells leads to activation of a cation conductance, calcium influx and blockade of delayed rectifying K channels. *Neuroscience,* **63**, 135–49.

Brambilla, R. and Klein, R. (1995). Telling axons where to grow: a role for Eph receptor tyrosine kinases in guidance. *Mol. and Cell. Neurosci.,* **6**, 487–95.

Bramham, C. R., Bacher-Svendsen, K., and Sarvey, J. M. (1997). LTP in the lateral perforant path is β-adrenergic receptor-dependent. *NeuroReport,* **8**, 719–24.

Bravarenko, N. I., Gusev, P. V., Balaban, P. M., and Voronin, L. L. (1995).

Postsynaptic induction of long-lasting facilitation in snail central neurones. *NeuroReport,* **6**, 1182–6.

Brorson, J. R., Sulit, R. A., and Zhang, H. (1997). Nitric oxide disrupts Ca^{2+} homeostasis in hippocampal neurons. *J. Neurochem.,* **68**, 95–105.

Brown, E. R. (1996). Voltage dependent Ca^{2+} release in invertebrate neurons. In: Annual meeting of the Society for Experimental Biology, University of Lancaster, Animal and Animal/Cell Abstracts, p. 11.

Buchholz, J., Nikkah, L., and Duckles, S. P. (1994). Age-related changes in the sensitivity of sympathetic nerves to altered extracellular calcium in tail arteries of F-344 rats. *Neurobiol. Aging,* **15**, 197–201.

Budd, S. L. and Nicholls, D. G. (1996). Mitochondria, calcium regulation, and acute glutamate excitotoxicity in cultured cerebellar granule cells. *J. Neurochem.,* **67**, 2282–91.

Burne, J. F. and Raff, M. C. (1997). Retinal ganglion cell axons drive the proliferation of astrocytes in the developing rodent optic nerve. *Neuron,* **18**, 223–30.

Cambray-Deakin, M. A., Foster, A. C., and Burgoyne, R. D. (1990). The expression of excitatory amino acid binding sites during neuritogenesis in the developing rat cerebellum. *Develop. Brain Res.,* **54**, 265–71.

Campbell, L. W., Hao, S.-Y., Thibault, O., Blalock, E. M., and Landsfield, P. W. (1996). Aging changes in voltage-gated calcium currents in hippocampal CA1 neurons. *J. Neurosci.,* **16**, 6286–95.

Carter, B. D. and Lewin, G. R. (1997). Neurotrophins live or let die: does $p75^{NTR}$ decide? *Neuron,* **18**, 187–90.

Castillo, P. E., Weiskopf, M. G., and Nicoll, R. A. (1994). The role of Ca^{2+} channels in hippocampal mossy fiber synaptic transmission and long-term potentiation. *Neuron,* **12**, 261–9.

Challacombe, J. F., Snow, D. M., and Letourneau, P. C. (1997). Dynamic microtubule ends are required for growth cone turning to avoid an inhibitory guidance cue. *J. Neurosci.,* **17**, 3085–95.

Chang, H. Y., Takei, K., Sydor, A. M., Born, T., Rusnack, F., and Jay, G. (1995). Asymmetric retraction of growth cone filopodia following focal inactivation of calcineurin. *Nature,* **376**, 686–90.

Chavis, P., Fagni, L., Lansman, J. B., and Bockaert, J. (1996). Functional coupling between ryanodine receptors and L-type calcium channels in neurons. *Nature,* **382**, 719–22.

Chiou, J.-Y. and Westhead, E. W. (1992). Okadaic acid, a protein phosphatase inhibitor, inhibits nerve growth factor-directed neurite outgrowth in PC12 cells. *J. Neurochem.,* **59**, 1963–6.

Chow, R. H., Klingauf, J., and Neher, E. (1994). Time course of Ca^{2+} concentration triggering exocytosis in neuroendocrine cells. *Proc. Natl Acad. Sci. USA,* **91**, 12765–9.

Christie, B. R., Magee, J. C., and Johnston, D. (1996). Dendritic calcium channels and hippocampal long-term depression. *Hippocampus,* **6**, 17–23.

Chung, J.-M., Huguenard, J. R., and Prince, D. A. (1993). Transient enhancement of low-threshold calcium current in thalamic relay neurons after corticotomy. *J. Neurophysiol.,* **70**, 20–7.

Cohan, C. S., Connor, J. A., and Kater, S. B. (1987). Electrically and chemically mediated increases in intracellular calcium in neuronal growth cones. *J. Neurosci.,* **7**, 3588–99.

Collingridge, G. L. (1987). The role of NMDA receptors in learning and memory. *Nature,* **330**, 604–5.

Connor, J. A., Miller, L. D. P., Petrozzino, J., and Muller, W. (1994). Calcium signalling in dendritic spines of hippocampal neurons. *J. Neurobiol.,* **25**, 234–42.

Corvalan, V., Cole, R., DeVillis, J., and Hagiwara, S. (1990). Neuronal modulation of calcium channel activity in cultured astrocytes. *Proc. Natl. Acad. Sci. USA,* **87**, 4345–8.

Coulter, D. A., Huguenard, J. R., and Prince, D. A. (1989). Calcium currents in rat thalamo cortical relay neurones: kinetic properties of the transient, low-threshold current. *J. Physiol. (London),* **414**, 587–604.

Coulter, D. A., Huguenard, J. R., and Prince, D. A. (1990). Differential effects of petit mal anticonvulsants and convulsants on thalamic neurones: calcium current reduction. *Br. J. Pharmacol.,* **100**, 800–6.

Cummings, J. A., Nicola, S. M., and Malenka R. C. (1994). Induction in the hippocampus of long-term potentiation (LTP) and long-term depression (LTD) in the presence of nitric oxide synthase inhibitors. *Neurosci. Lett.,* **176**, 110–14.

Cummings, J. A., Mulkey, R. M., Nicoll, R. A., and Malenka, R. C. (1996). Ca^{2+} signalling requirements for long-term depression in the hippocampus. *Neuron,* **16**, 825–33.

Dai, Z. and Peng, H. B. (1993). Elevation in presynaptic Ca^{2+} level accompanying initial nerve-muscle contact in tissue culture. *Neuron,* **10**, 827–37.

Dailey, M. and Smith, S. J. (1996). The dynamics of dendritic structure in developing hippocampal slices. *J. Neurosci.,* **16**, 2983–94.

Dani, J. W., Chernjavsky, A., and Smith, S. J. (1992). Neuronal activity triggers calcium waves in hippocampal astrocyte networks. *Neuron,* **8**, 429–40.

Das, N. and Ghosh, S. (1996). The effect of age on calcium dynamics in rat brain in vivo. *Mech. Ageing Dev.,* **88**, 17–24.

Davenport, R. W., Dou, P., Mills, L. R., and Kater, S. B. (1996). Distinct calcium signalling within neuronal growth cones and filopodia. *J. Neurobiol.,* **31**, 1–15.

Dawson, V. L., Dawson, T. M., London, G. D., Bredt, D. S., and Snyder, S. H. (1991). Nitric oxide mediates glutamate neurotoxicity in primary cortical cultures. *Proc. Natl. Acad. Sci. USA,* **88**, 6368–71.

Debanne, D. and Thompson, S. M. (1994). Calcium: a trigger for long-term depression and potentiation in the hippocampus. *News Physiol. Sci.,* **9**, 256–60.

Debanne, D. and Thompson, S. M. (1996). Associative long-term depression in the hippocampus in vitro. *Hippocampus,* **6**, 9–16.

De Jong, G. I., Naber, P. A., Van der Zee, E. A., Thompson, L. T., Disterhoft, J. F., and Luiten, P. G. M. (1996). Age-related loss of calcium binding proteins in rabbit hippocampus. *Neurobiol. Aging,* **17**, 459–65.

De Koninck, Y. and Mody, I. (1996). The effects of raising intracellular calcium on synaptic $GABA_A$ receptor-channels. *Neuropharmacology.* **35**, 1365–74.

Delaney, K. R., Zucker, R. S., and Tank, D. W. (1989) Calcium in motor nerve terminals associated with posttetanic potentiation. *J. Neurosci.,* **9**, 3558–67.

DeLorme, E. M., Rabe, C. S., and McGee, R., Jr (1988). Regulation of the number of functional voltage-sensitive Ca^{++} channels on PC12 cells by chronic changes in membrane potential. *J. Pharmacol. Exp. Ther.,* **244**, 838–43.

Denk, W., Sugimori, M., and Llinas, R. (1995). Two types of calcium response limited to single spines in cerebellar Purkinje cells. *Proc. Natl. Acad. Sci. USA,* **92**, 8279–82.

Desarmenien, M. G., Clendening, B., and Spitzer, N. C. (1993) In vivo development of voltage-dependent ionic currents in embryonic *Xenopus* spinal neurons. *J. Neurosci.,* **13**, 2575–81.

Destexhe, A., Contreras, D., Steriade, M., Sejnowski, T. J., and Huguenard, J. R. (1996). In vivo, in vitro, and computational analysis of dendritic calcium currents in thalamic reticular neurons. *J. Neurosci.,* **16**, 169–85.

Disterhoft, J. F., Moyer, J. R. and Thompson, L. T. (1994). The calcium rationale in aging. Alzheimer's disease: evidence from an animal model of normal aging. *Ann. New York Acad. Sci.,* **747**, 382–406.

Disterhoft, J. F., Thompson, L. T., Moyer, J. R., Jr, and Mogul, D. J. (1996). Calcium-dependent afterhyperpolarization and learning in young and aging hippocampus. *Life Sci.,* **59**, 413–20.

D'Mello, S. R., Borodezt, K., and Soloff, S. P. (1997). Insulin-like growth factor and potassium depolarization maintain neuronal survival by distinct pathways: possible involvement of PI 3-kinase in IGF-1 signalling. *J. Neurosci.,* **17**, 1548–60.

Doherty, P. and Walsh, F. S. (1991). The contrasting roles of N-CAM and N-cadherin as neurite outgrowth-promoting molecules. *J. Cell Sci.,* Suppl. 15, 13–21.

Doherty, P., Rowett, L. H., Moore, S. E., Mann, D. A., and Walsh, F. S. (1991). Neurite outgrowth in response to transfected N-CAM and N-cadherin reveals fundamental differences in neuronal responsiveness to CAMs. *Neuron,* **6**, 247–58.

Doroshenko, P. A., Kostyuk, P. G., and Martynyuk, A. E. (1982). Intracellular metabolism of adenosine 3',5'-cyclic monophosphate and calcium inward current in perfused neurones of *Helix pomatia*. *Neuroscience,* **9**, 2125–34.

Doyle, C. A., Cullen, W. K., Rowan, M. J., and Amwyl, R. (1997). Low-frequency stimulation induces homosynaptic depotentiation but not long-term depression of synaptic transmission in the adult anaesthetized and awake rta hippocampus in vivo. *Neuroscience,* **77**, 75–85.

Dubinsky, J. M. (1993). Examination of the role of calcium in neuronal death. *Ann. New York Acad. Sci.,* **679**, 34–42.

Duckles, S. P., Tsai, H., and Buchholz, J. N. (1996). Evidence for decline in intracellular calcium buffering in adrenergic nerves of aged rats. *Life Sci.,* **58**, 2029–35.

Dudek, S. M. and Bear, M. F. (1992). Homosynaptic long-term depression in area CA1 of hippocampus and effects of *N*-methyl-D-aspartate receptor blockade. *Proc. Natl. Acad. Sci. USA,* **89**, 4363–7.

Eccles, J. C. (1964). *The physiology of synapses.* Springer, Heidelberg.

Eckert, A., Hartmann, H., Förstl, H., and Müller, W. E. (1994). Alterations of intracellular calcium regulation during aging and Alzheimer's disease in nonneuronal cells. *Life Sci.,* **55**, 2019–29.

Eilers, J., Callewaert, G., Armstrong, C. and Konnerth, A. (1995). Calcium signalling in a narrow somatic submembrane shell during synaptic activity in cerebellar Purkinje neurones. *Proc. Natl. Acad. Sci. USA,* **92**, 10272–6.

Eilers, J., Plant, T. and Konnerth, A. (1996). Localized calcium signalling and neuronal integration in cerebellar Purkinje neurones. *Cell Calcium*, **20**, 215–26.

Fedulova, S. A., Kostyuk, P. G., and Veselovsky, N. S. (1985). Two types of calcium channels in the somatic membrane of newborn rat dorsal root ganglion neurones. *J. Physiol. (London),* **359**, 431–46.

Fedulova, S. A., Kostyuk, P. G., and Veselovsky, N. S. (1986). Changes in ionic mechanisms of electrical excitability of the somatic membrane of rat dorsal root ganglion neurons during ontogenesis. Correlation between inward current densities. *Neurophysiology (Kiev),* **18**, 581–6 (English edition).

Fedulova, S. A., Kostyuk, P. G., and Veselovsky, N. S. (1994). Comparative analysis of ionic currents in the somatic membrane of sensory neurons from embryonic and newborn rats. *Neuroscience,* **58**, 341–6.

Ferroni, A., Galli, A., and Mazzanti, M. (1996). Functional role of low-voltage-activated dihydropyridine-sensitive Ca channels during the action potential in adult rat sensory neurones. *Pfluegers Arch.,* **431**, 954–63.

Finkbeiner, S. M. (1993). Glial calcium. *Glia,* **9**, 83–104.

Franklin, J. L. and Johnson, E. M. (1992). Suppression of programmed neuronal death by sustained elevation of cytoplasmic calcium. *TINS,* **15**, 501–7.

Franklin, J. L. and Johnson, E. M. (1994). Elevated intracellular calcium blocks programmed neuronal death. *Ann. New York Acad. Sci.,* **747**, 195–204.

Franklin, J. L., Sanz-Rodriguez, C., Juhasz, A., Deckwerth, T. L., and Johnson, E. M., Jr (1995). Chronic depolarization prevents programmed death of sympathetic neurons in vitro but does not support growth: requirement for Ca2+ influx but not Trk activation. *J. Neurosci.,* **15**, 643–64.

Friel, D. D. and Tsien, R. W. (1994). An FCCP-sensitive Ca^{2+} store in bullfrog sympathetic neurons and its participation in stimulus-evoked changes in $[Ca^{2+}]_i$. *J. Neurosci.,* **14**, 4007–24.

Fukunaga, K., Muller, D., and Miyamoto, E. (1996). CaM Kinase II in long-term potentiation. *Neurochem. Int.,* **28**, 343–58.

Funayama, M., Goto, K., and Kondo, H. (1996). Cloning and expression localization of cDNA for rat homolog of TRP protein, a possible store-operated calcium (Ca^{2+}) channel. *Mol. Brain Res.,* **43**, 259–66.

Funte, L. R. and Haydon, P. G. (1993). Synaptic target contact enhances presynaptic calcium influx by activating cAMP-dependent protein kinase during synaptogenesis. *Neuron,* **10**, 1069–78.

Gerasimenko, O. V., Gerasimenko, J. V., Tepikin, A. V., and Petersen, O. H. (1995). ATP-dependent accumulation and inositol triphosphate- or cyclic ADP-ribose-mediated release of Ca^{2+} from the nuclear envelop. *Cell,* **80**, 439–44.

Gerasimenko, O. V., Gerasimenko, J. V., Tepikin, A. V., and Petersen, O. H. (1996*a*). Calcium transport pathways in the nucleus. *Pfluegers Arch.,* **432**, 1–6.

Gerasimenko, O.V., Gerasimenko, J.V., Belan, P.V. and Petersen, O. H. (1996*b*). Inositol triphosphate and cyclic ADP-ribose-mediated release of Ca^{2+} from single isolated pancreatic zymogen granules. *Cell,* **84**, 473–80.

Gill, D. L., Waldron, R. T., Rys-Sikora, K. E., Ufret-Vincenty, C. A., Graber, M. N., Favre, C. J., *et al.* (1996). Calcium pools, calcium entry, and cell growth. *Biosci. Rep.,* **16**, 139–57.

Ginty, D. D. (1997). Calcium regulation of gene expression: isn't that spatial? *Neuron,* **18**, 183–6.

Giulian, D. (1993). Reactive glia as rivals in regulatory neuronal survival. *Glia,* **7**, 102–10.

Glazewski, S., Skangiel-Kramska, J., and Kossut, M. (1993). Development of NMDA receptor-channel complex and L-type calcium channels in mouse hippocampus. *J. Neurosci.,* **35**, 199–206.

Glitsch, M., Llano, I., and Marty, A. (1996). Glutamate as a candidate retrograde messenger at interneurone–Purkinje cell synapses of rat cerebellum. *J. Physiol. (London)*, **497**, 531–7.

Glowinski, J., Marin, P., Tence, M., Stella, N., Giaume, C., and Premont, J. (1994). Glial receptors and their intervention in astrocyto–astrocytic and astrocyto–neuronal interactions. *Glia,* **11**, 201–8.

Gomez, J.-P., Potreau, D., Branka, J.-E., and Raymond, G. (1994). Developmental changes in Ca2+ currents from newborn rat cardiomyocytes in primary culture. *Pfluegers Arch.,* **428**, 241–9.

Gomez, T. M., Snow, D. M., and Letourneau, P. C. (1995). Characterization of spontaneous calcium transients in nerve growth cones and their effect on growth cone migration. *Neuron,* **14**, 1233–46.

Gottmann, K. J., Rohrer, H., and Lux, H. D. (1991). Distribution of Ca^{2+} and Na^{+} conductance during neuronal differentiation of chick DRG precursor cells. *J. Neurosci.,* **11**, 3371–8.

Gribkoff, V. K. and Lum-Ragan, J. T. (1992). Evidence for nitric-oxide-synthase inhibitor-sensitive and insensitive hippocampal synaptic potentiation. *J. Neurophysiol.,* **68**, 639–42.

Gruol, D. L. and Parsons, K. L. (1994). Chronic exposure to alcohol during development alters the calcium currents of cultured cerebellar Purkinje neurons. *Brain Res.,* **634**, 283–90.

Gu, X. N. and Spitzer, N. C. (1997). Breaking the code: regulation of neuronal differentiation by spontaneous calcium transients. *Dev. Neurosci.,* **19**, 33–41.

Haimovich, B., Tanaka, J. C., and Barchi, R. L. (1986). Developmental appearance of sodium channel subtypes in rat skeletal muscle cultures. *J. Neurochem.,* **47**, 1148–53.

Harris, E. W. and Cotman, C. W. (1986). Long-term potentiation of guinea-pig mossy fiber responses is not blocked by *N*-methyl-D-aspartate antagonists. *Neurosci. Lett.,* **70**, 132–7.

Harris, G. L., Henderson, L. P., and Spitzer, H. C. (1988). Changes in densities and kinetics of delayed rectifier potassium channels during neuronal differentiation. *Neuron,* **1**, 739–50.

Harrold, J., Ritchie, J., Nicholls, D., Smith, W., Bowman, D., and Pocock, J. (1997). The development of Ca2+ channels responses and their coupling to exocytosis in cultured cerebellar granule cells. *Neuroscience,* **77**, 683–94.

Hartell, N. A. (1996). Inhibition of cGMP breakdown promotes the induction of cerebellar long-term depression. *J. Neurosci.,* **16**, 2881–90.

Hartmann, H., Eckert, A., and Müller, W. E. (1993*a*). Aging enhances the calcium sensitivity of central neurons of the mouse as an adaptive response to reduced free intracellular calcium. *Neurosci. Lett.,* **152**, 181–4.

Hartmann, H., Eckert, A., and Müller, W. E. (1993*b*). β-Amyloid protein amplifies calcium signalling in central neurons from the adult mouse. *Biochem. Biophys. Res. Commun.,* **16**, 1216–20.

Hartmann, H., Eckert, A., and Müller, W. E. (1994). Disturbances of the neuronal calcium homeostasis in the aging nervous system. *Life Sci.,* **55**, 2011–18.

Hartmann, H., Eckert, A., Velbinger, K., Rewsin, M., and Müller, W. E. (1996*a*). Down-regulation of free intracellular calcium in dissociated brain cells of aged mice and rats. *Life Sci.,* **59**, 435–49.

Hartmann, H., Velbinger, K., Eckert, A., and Müller, W. E. (1996). Region-specific downregulation of free intracellular calcium in the aged rat brain. *Neurobiol. Aging,* **17**, 557–63.

Hashimoto, T., Ishii, T., and Ohmori, H. (1996*b*). Release of Ca^{2+} is the crucial step for the potentiation of IPSCs in the cultured cerebellar Purkinje cells of the rat. *J. Physiol. (London),* **497**, 611–27.

Hegarty, J. L., Kay, A. R., and Green, S. H. (1997). Trophic support of cultured spiral ganglion neurons by depolarization exceeds and is additive with that by neurotrophins or cAMP and requires elevation of $[Ca^{2+}]_i$ within a set range. *J. Neurosci.,* **17**, 1959–70.

Hertz, L. (1978). An intense potassium uptake into astrocytes, further enhancement by high concentrations of potassium and possible involvement in potassium homeostasis at the cellular level. *Brain Res.,* **145**, 202–8.

Hillman, D. E., Chen, S., Bing, R., Penniston, J. T. and Llinas, R. (1996). Ultrastructural localization of the plasmalemmal calcium pump in cerebellar neurons. *Neuroscience*, **72**, 315–24.

Himmelseher, S., Pfenniger, E., and Georgieff, M. (1997). Effects of basic fibroblast growth factor on hippocampal neurons after axonal injury. *J. Trauma Injury Infect. Crit. Care,* **42**, 659–64.

Hockberger, P. E., Tseng, H.-Y., and Connor, J. A. (1987). Immuno-cytochemical and electrophysiological differentiation of rat cerebellar granule cells in explant cultures. *J. Neurosci.,* **7**, 1370–83.

Hockberger, P. E., Tseng, H.-Y., and Connor, J. A. (1989). Development of rat cerebellar Purkinje cells: electrophysiological properties following acute isolation and in long-term culture. *J. Neurosci.,* **9**, 2258–71.

Holliday, J. and Spitzer, N. C. (1990). Spontaneous calcium influx and its roles in differentiation of spinal neurons in culture. *Dev. Biol.,* **141**, 13–23.

Holliday, J. and Spitzer, N. C. (1993). Calcium regulates neuronal differentiation both directly and via co-cultured myocytes. *J. Neurobiol.,* **24**, 506–14.

Holliday, J., Adams, R. J., Sejnowski, T. J., and Spitzer, N. C. (1991). Calcium-induced release of calcium regulates differentiation of cultured spinal neurons. *Neuron,* **7**, 787–96.

Holliday, J., Parsons, K., Curry, J., Lee, S. Y., and Gruol, D. L. (1995).

Cerebellar granule neurons develop elevated calcium responses when treated with interleukin-6 in culture. *Brain Res.,* **673**, 141–8.

Holmes, W. R. (1990). Is the function of dendritic spines to concentrate calcium? *Brain Res.,* **519**, 338–42.

Holzwarth, J. A., Gibbons, S. J., Brorson, J. R., Philipson, L. H., and Niuller, R. J. (1994). Glutamate receptor agonists stimulate divers calcium responses in different types of cultured rat cortical glial cells. *J. Neurosci.,* **14**, 1879–91.

Huang, C.-M., Tsay, K.-E., and Kao, L.-S. (1996). Role of Ca^{2+} in differentiation mediated by nerve growth factor and dibutyryl cyclic AMP in PC12 cells. *J. Neurochem.,* **67**, 530–9.

Huang, L. Q., Rowan, M. J., and Anwyl, R. (1997). mGluR II agonist inhibition of LTP induction, and mGluR II antagonist inhibition of LTD induction, in the dentate gyrus in vitro. *NeuroReport,* **8**, 687–93.

Huang, W. C. and Chueh, S. H. (1996). Calcium mobilization from the intracellular mitochondrial and nonmitochondrial stores of the rat cerebellum. *Brain Res.,* **718**, 151–8.

Huber, K. M., Mauk, M. D., and Kelly, P. T. (1995). LTP induced by activation of voltage-dependent Ca^{2+} channels requires protein kinase activity. *NeuroReport,* **6**, 1281–84.

Hubschl, T., Madeja, M., Musshoff, U., and Spechmann, E. J. (1997). Membrane currents elicited by the organic calcium channel blocker verapamil in native and rat-brain RNA injected oocytes of *Xenopus laevis*. *Arzneimittelforschung,* **47**, 1–5.

Huguenard, J. P. (1996). Low-threshold calcium currents in central nervous system neurons. *Annu. Rev. Physiol.,* **58**, 329–48.

Huguenard, J. P. and Prince, D. A. (1992). A novel T-type current underlies prolonged Ca^{2+}-dependent burst firing in GABAergic neurons of rat thalamic reticular neurons. *J. Neurosci.,* **12**, 3804–17.

Humbert, J.-P., Matter, N., Artault, J.-C., Koeppler, P., and Malviya, A. N. (1996). Inositol 1,4,5-triphosphate receptor is located to the inner nuclear membrane indicating regulation of nuclear calcium signalling by inositol 1,4,5-triphosphate. *J. Biol. Chem.,* **271**, 478–85.

Hutcheon, B., Miura, R. M., Yarom, Y., and Puil, E. (1994). Low-threshold calcium current and resonance in thalamic neurons: a model of frequency preference. *J. Neurophysiol.,* **71**, 583–94.

Ikegava, Y., Yoshida, M., Saito, H., and Nishiyama, N. (1997). Epileptic activity prevents synapse formation of hippocampal mossy fibers via L-type calcium channel activation in vitro. *J. Pharmacol. Exp. Ther.,* **280**, 471–6.

Improta, T., Salvatore, A. M., Di Luzio, A., Romeo, G., Coccia, E. M., and Calissano, P. (1988) IFN-γ-facilitates NGF-induced neuronal differentiation in PC12 cells. *Exp. Cell Res.,* **179**, 1–9.

Isaev, D. S., Eremin, A. V., and Tarasenko, A. N. (1997). Developmental changes in expression of low-voltage-activated Ca^{2+} channels in rat cortical and thalamic neurons. *Neurophysiology (Kiev)*, **29**, 368 (English edition).

Izumi, Y. and Zorumski, C. F. (1993). Nitric oxide and long-term synaptic depression in the rat hippocampus. *NeuroReport*, **4**, 1131–4.

Janigro, D., Gasparini, S., D'Ambrosio, R., McKhann, G., and DiFrancesco, D. (1997). Reduction of K^+ uptake in glia prevents long-term depression maintenance and causes epileptiform activity. *J. Neurosci.*, **17**, 2813–24.

Jessell, T. M. and Kansel, E. R. (1993). Synaptic transmission: a bidirectional and self-modifiable form of cell–cell communication. *Neuron*, **10**, 1–30.

Jimenez, C., Gireldez, F., Represa, J., and Garcia-Diaz, J. F. (1997). Calcium currents in dissociated cochlear neurons from the chick embryo and their modification by neurotrophin-3. *Neuroscience*, **77**, 673–82.

Johnson, E. M., Jr and Deckwerth, T. L. (1993). Molecular mechanisms of developmental neuronal death. *Annu. Rev. Neurosci.*, **16**, 31–46.

Johnson, F., Hohmann, S. E., DiStefano, P. S., and Bottjer, S. W. (1997). Neurotrophins suppers apoptosis induced by deafferentation of an avian motor-cortical region. *J. Neurosci.*, **17**, 2101–11.

Kaczmarek, L., Kossut, M., and Skangiel-Kramska, J. (1997). Glutamate receptors in cortical plasticity: molecular and cellular biology. *Physiol. Rev.*, **77**, 217–55.

Kamiya, H. and Zucker, R. S. (1994). Residual Ca^{2+} and short-term synaptic plasticity. *Nature*, **371**, 603–6.

Kaneda, M., Wakamori, M., Ito, C., and Akaike, N. (1990). Low-threshold calcium current in isolated Purkinje cell bodies of rat cerebellum. *J. Neurophysiol.*, **63**, 1046–51.

Kang, Y. and Kitai, S. T. (1993). A whole cell patch-clamp study on the pacemaker potential in dopaminergic neurons of rat substantia nigra compacta. *Neurosci. Res.*, **18**, 209–221.

Kano, M., Satoh, R., and Nakabayashi, Y. (1991). Developmental changes in voltage-dependent calcium and sodium channels during differentiation of embryonic chick skeletal muscle cells in cultures. *Biomed. Res.* **12** (Suppl.), 197–8.

Kano, M., Garaschuk, O., Verkhratsky, A., and Konnerth, A. (1995). Ryanodine receptor-mediated intracellular calcium release in rat cerebellar Purkinje neurones. *J. Physiol. (London)*, **487**, 1–16.

Karst, H., Joels, M., and Wadman, J. (1993). Low-threshold calcium current in dendrites of the adult rat hippocampus. *Neurosci. Lett.*, **164**, 154–8.

Kasono, K. and Hirano, T. (1995*a*). Critical role of postsynaptic calcium in cerebellar long-term depression. *NeuroReport*, **6**, 17–20.

Kasono, K. and Hirano, T. (1995*b*) Involvement of inositol triphosphate in cerebellar long-term depression. *NeuroReport*, **6**, 569–72.

Katsuki, H., Izumi, Y., and Zorumski, C. F. (1997). Removal of extracellular calcium after conditioning stimulation disrupts long-term potentiation in the CA1 region of rat hippocampal slices. *Neuroscience,* **76**, 1113–19.

Katz, E., Ferro, P. A., Weisz, G., and Uchitel, O. D. (1996). Calcium channels involved in synaptic transmission at the mature and regenerating mouse neuromuscular junction. *J. Physiol. (London)* **497**, 687–97.

Kawano, S. and DeHaan, R. L. (1991). Developmental changes in the calcium currents in embryonic ventricular myocytes. *J. Membr. Biol.,* **120**, 17–28.

Kawasaki, K., Czeh, G., and Somjen, G. G. (1988). Prolonged exposure to high potassium concentration results in irreversible loss of synaptic transmission in hippocampal tissue slices. *Brain Res.,* **457**, 322–9.

Kerr, D. S., Campbell, L. W., Thibault, O., and Landfield, P. W. (1992) Hippocampal glucocorticoid receptor activation enhances voltage-dependent Ca^{2+} conductances; relevance to brain aging. *Proc. Natl. Acad. Sci. USA,* **89**, 8527–31.

Kettenmann, H. and Ransom, B. R. (1988). Electrical coupling between astrocytes and between oligodendrocytes studied on mammalian cell culture. *Glia,* **1**, 64–73.

Kettenmann, H., Kirischuk, S., and Verkhratsky, A. (1994). Calcium signalling in oligodendrocytes. *Neurophysiology (Kiev),* **26**, 21–5 (English edition).

Keynes, R. and Cook, G. M. W. (1995). Axon guidance molecules. *Cell,* **83**, 161–9.

Kirischuk, S. I. (1996). *Mechanisms of calcium signalling in glial cells from central nervous system.* Dissertation for D. Sc. degree, Bogomoletz Institute of Physiology, Kiev, pp. 24–6.

Kirischuk, S. and Verkhratsky, A. (1996). Calcium homeostasis in aged neurones. *Life Sci.,* **59**, 451–9.

Kirischuk, S., Pronchuk, N., and Verkhratsky, A. (1992). Measurements of intracellular calcium in sensory neurons of adult and old rats. *Neuroscience,* **50**, 947–51.

Kirischuk, S., Voitenko, N., Kettenmann, H., and Verkhratsky, A. (1994). Mechanisms of cytoplasmic calcium signalling in cerebellar Bergmann glial cells. *Neurophysiology (Kiev),* **26**, 341–3 (English edition).

Kirischuk, S., Moller, T., Voitenko, N., Kettenmann, H., and Verkhratsky, A. (1995*a*). ATP-triggered calcium mobilization in cerebellar Bergmann glial cells. *J. Neurosci.,* **15**, 7861–71.

Kirischuk, S., Scherer, J., Müller, T., Kettenmann, H., and Verkhratsky, A. (1995*b*). Subcellular heterogeneity of voltage-gated Ca^{2+} channels in cells of oligodendrocyte lineage. *Glia,* **13**, 1–12.

Kirischuk, S., Scherer, J., Kettenmann, H., and Verkhratsky, A. (1995*c*).

Activation of P_2-purinoreceptors triggered Ca^{2+} release from $InsP_3$-sensitive internal stores in mammalian oligodendrocytes. *J. Physiol. (London)* **483**, 41–57.

Kirischuk, S., Matiash, V., Kulik, A., Voitenko, N., Kostyuk, P., and Verkhratsky, A. (1996*a*). Activation of P_2-purino, α_1-adreno and H_1-histamine receptors triggers cytoplasmic calcium signalling in cerebellar Purkinje neurons. *Neuroscience,* **73**, 643–7.

Kirischuk, S., Tuchick, S., Verkhratsky, A., and Kettenmann, H. (1996*b*). Epinephrine and histamine-induced Ca^{2+} signalling in Bergmann glia. *Eur. J. Neurosci.,* **8**, 1198–1208.

Kirischuk, S., Voitenko, N., Kostyuk, P., and Verkhratsky, A. (1996*c*). Age-associated changes of cytoplasmic calcium homeostasis in cerebellar granule neurones in situ: investigation on thin cerebellar slice. *Exp. Gerontol.,* **31**, 475–87.

Klein, M., Hochner, B., and Kandel, E. R. (1986). Facilitatory transmitters and cAMP can modulate accommodation as well as transmitter release in *Aplysia* sensory neurons: evidence fore parallel processing in a single cell. *Proc. Natl. Acad. Sci. USA,* **83**, 7994–8.

Klingauf, J. and Neher, E. (1997). Modeling buffered Ca^{2+} diffusion near the membrane: implications for secretion in neuroendocrine cells. *Biophys. J.,* **72**, 674–90.

Klishin, A., Lozovaya, N., and Krishtal, O. (1994). Persistently enhanced ration of NMDA and non-NMDA components in rat hippocampal EPSC after block of A_1 adenosine receptors at increased $[Ca^{2+}]_o/[Mg^{2+}]_o$. *Neurosci. Lett.,* **179**, 132–6.

Klishin, A., Lozovaya, N., and Krishtal, O. (1995). A_1-adenosine receptors differentially regulate the *N*-methyl-d-aspartate and non-*N*-methyl-d-aspartate receptor-mediated components of hippocampal excitatory postsynaptic current in a Ca^{2+}/Mg^{2+} -dependent manner. *Neuroscience,* **65**, 947–53.

Klishin, A., Tsintsadze, T., Lozovaya, N., and Krishtal, O. A. (1995). Latent *N*-methyl-d-aspartate receptors in the recurrent excitatory pathway between hippocampal CA1 pyramidal neurons: Ca^{++}-dependent activation by blocking A_1-adenosine receptors. *Proc. Natl. Acad. Sci. USA,* **92**, 12431–5.

Knoops, B. and Octave, J.-N. (1997). α_1-tubulin mRNA level is increased during neurite outgrowth of NG 108–15 cells but not during neurite outgrowth inhibition by CNS myelin. *NeuroReport,* **8**, 795–8.

Kobrinsky, E. M., Pearson, H. A., and Dolphin, A. C. (1994). Low- and high-voltage-activated calcium channel currents and their modulation in the dorsal root ganglion cell line ND7–23. *Neuroscience,* **58**, 539–52.

Koike, T. (1983). Nerve growth factor-induced neurite outgrowth of rat pheochromo cytoma PC12 cells: dependence on extracellular Mg^{2+} and Ca^{2+}. *Brain Res.*, **289**, 293–304.

Koizumi, S., Kitaoka, Y., Inoue, K., Kohzuma, M., Niwa, M., and Taniyama, K. (1995). Contribution of L-type Ca^{2+} channels to long-term enhancement of high K^{+}-evoked release of dopamine from rat striatal slices. *Neurosci. Lett.*, **187**, 123–6.

Kojima, M. and Sperelakis, N. (1985). Development of slow Ca^{2+}–Na^{+} channels during organ culture of young embryonic chick hearts. *J. Dev. Physiol.*, **7**, 355–63.

Komatsu, Y. (1994). Plasticity of excitatory synaptic transmission in kitten visual cortex depends on voltage-dependent Ca^{++} channels but not on NMDA receptors. *Neurosci. Res.*, **20**, 209–12.

Komatsu, Y. (1996). $GABA_B$ receptors, monoamine receptors, and postsynaptic inositol tris-phosphate-induced Ca^{2+} release are involved in the induction of long-term potentiation at visual cortical inhibitory synapses. *J. Neurosci.*, **16**, 6342–52.

Komatsu, Y. and Iwakiri, M. (1992). Low-threshold Ca^{2+} channels mediate induction of long-term potentiation in kitten visual cortex. *J. Neurophysiol.*, **67**, 401–10.

Komura, H. and Rakic, P. (1992). Selective role of N-type calcium channels in neuronal migration. *Science*, **257**, 806–9.

Komura, H. and Rakic, P. (1993). Modulation of neuronal migration by NMDA receptors. *Science*, **260**, 95–7.

Konnerth, A. (1995). Cellular mechanisms of synaptic plasticity in cerebellar Purkinje cells. *J. Neurochem.*, **65**, Suppl. S139.

Kostyuk, E. P. and Shmigol, A. V. (1995). Effect of insulin and nimodipin on calcium signals in murine primary afferent neurons with experimental diabetes. *Neurophysiology, (Kiev)* **27**, 270–5 (English edition).

Kostyuk, E. P., Pronchuk, N., and Shmigol, A. V. (1995). Calcium signal prolongation in sensory neurons of mice with experimental diabetes. *NeuroReport*, **6**, 1010–12.

Kostyuk, P. G. (1992). *Calcium ions in nerve cell function.* Oxford University Press.

Kostyuk, P. G. and Lukyanetz, E. A. (1993). Mechanisms of antagonistic action of internal Ca^{2+} on serotonin-induced potentiation of Ca^{2+} currents in *Helix* neurones. *Pfluegers Arch.*, **424**, 73–83.

Kostyuk, P. G. and Lukyanetz, E. A. (1994). Intracellular mechanisms of calcium channel modulation by serotonin in identified *Helix pomatia* neurons. *Netherlands J. Zool.*, **44**, 512–23.

Kostyuk, P. G. and Shmigol, A. V. (1997). Intracellular stores and calcium signalling in mammalian sensory neurones. *Bioelectrochem. Bioenerg.*, **42**, 197–205.

Kostyuk, P. G. and Verkhratsky, A. N. (1995). *Calcium signalling in the nervous system.* Wiley, Chichester.

Kostyuk, P. G., Krishtal, O. A., Pidoplichko, V. I., and Veselovsky, N. S. (1978). Ionic currents in the neuroblastoma cell membrane. *Neuroscience,* **3**, 327–32.

Kostyuk, P. G., Fedulova, S. A., and Veselovsky, N. S. (1986). Changes in ionic mechanisms of electrical excitability of the somatic membrane of rat dorsal root ganglion neurons during ontogenesis: distribution of ionic channels of inward currents. *Neurophysiology (Kiev)* **18**, 575–80 (English edition).

Kostyuk, P. G., Lukyanetz, E. A., and Doroshenko, P. A. (1992). Effects of serotonin and cAMP on calcium currents in different neurones of *Helix pomatia. Pfluegers Arch.,* **420**, 9–15.

Kostyuk, P. G., Pronchuk, N. F., Savchenko, A. N., and Verkhratsky, A. N. (1993). Calcium currents in aged dorsal root ganglion neurones. *J. Physiol. (London),* **461**, 467–83.

Kristian, T., Ouyang, Y., and Siesjö, B. K. (1996). Calcium-induced neuronal cell death in vivo and in vitro: are the pathophysiologic mechanisms different? In: *Advances in neurology, Vol. 71, Cellular and molecular mechanisms in ischemic brain damage,* (ed. B. K. Siesjö and T. Wieloch), pp. 107–18. Lippincott-Raven, Philadelphia.

Krzywkowski, P., Potter, B., Billard, J. M., Dutar, P., and Lamour, Y. (1996). Synaptic mechanisms and calcium binding proteins in the aged rat brain. *Life Sci.,* **59**, 421–28.

Lampe, P. A., Cornbrooks, E. B., Juhasz, A., Johnson, E. M., Jr, and Franklin, J. L. (1995). Suppression of programmed neuronal death by a thapsigagrin-induced Ca^{2+} influx. *J. Neurobiol.,* **26**, 205–12.

Landfield, P. W. (1996). Aging-related increase in hippocampal calcium channels. *Life Sci.,* **59**, 399–404.

Landfield, P. W., Thibault, O., Mazzanti, M. L., Porter, N. M., and Kerr, D. S. (1992). Mechanisms of neuronal death in brain aging and Alzheimer's disease: role of endocrine-mediated calcium dyshomeastasis. *J. Neurobiol.,* **23**, 1247–60.

Larrabee, M. G. and Bronk, W. (1947). Prolonged facilitation of synaptic excitation in sympathetic ganglia. *J. Neurophysiol.,* **10**, 139–54.

Lee, S. H., Kim, W. T., Cornell-Bell, A. H., and Sontheimer, H. (1994). Astrocytes exhibit regional specificity in gar-junction coupling. *Glia,* **11**, 315–325.

Leinekugel, X., Medina, I., Khalilov, I., Ben-Ari, Y., and Khazipov, R. (1997). Ca^{2+} oscillations mediated by the synergistic excitatory action of $GABA_A$ and NMDA receptors in the neonatal hippocampus. *Neuron,* **18**, 243–55.

Lewis, D. L., de Aizpurua, H. J., and Rausch, D. M. (1993). Enhanced expression of Ca^{2+} channels by nerve growth factor and the v-src oncogene in rat phaeochromocytoma cells. *J. Physiol. (London),* **465**, 325–42.

Liebermann, D. and Sachs, L. (1978). Nuclear control of neurite induction in neuroblastoma cells. *Exp. Cell Res.,* **113**, 383–90.

Lin, X. Y. and Glanzman, D. L. (1996). Long-term depression of *Aplysia* sensorimotor synapses in cell culture: inductive role of a rise in postsynaptic calcium. *J. Neurophysiol.,* **76**, 2111–14.

Lin, Y. Q., Brain, K. L., Nichol, K. A., and Bennett, M. R. (1996). Vesicle-associated proteins and calcium in nerve terminals of chick ciliary ganglion during development of facilitation. *J. Physiol. (London),* **497**, 639–56.

Lisman, J. (1989). A mechanism for the Hebb and the anti-Hebb processes underlying learning and memory. *Proc. Natl. Acad. Sci. USA,* **86**, 9574–8

Liu, H., Felix, R., Gurnett, C. A., De Waard, M., Witcher, D. R., and Campbell, K. P. (1996). Expression and subunit interaction of voltage-dependent Ca^{++} channels in PC12 cells. *J. Neurosci.,* **16**, 7557–65.

Llinas, R., Sugimori, M, and Silver, R. B. (1992). Microdomains of high calcium concentration in a presynaptic terminal. *Science,* **256**, 677–9.

Lloyd, D. P. C. (1949). Post-tetanic potentiation of responses in mono-synaptic pathways of the spinal cord. *J. Gen. Physiol.,* **33**, 147–70.

Lozovaya, N. and Klee, M. R. (1995). Phorbol diacetate differentially regulates the *N*-methyl-d-aspartate (NMDA) and non-NMDA receptor mediated components of the rat hippocampal excitatory postsynaptic currents. *Neurosci. Lett.,* **189**, 101–4.

Lukyanetz, E. A. (1997). Evidence for colocalization of calcineurin and calcium channels in dorsal root ganglion neurons. *Neuroscience,* **78**, 625–8.

Lukyanetz, E. A. and Sotkis, A. V. (1996). Serotonin-induced changes in the activity of single Ca^{2+} channels in *Helix pomatia* neurons. *Neurophysiology (Kiev),* **28**, 103–10 (English edition).

Lukyanetz, E. A. and Sotkis, A. V. (1996). Characterization of single K^+ channels in *Helix pomatia* neurons. *Neurophysiology (Kiev),* **28**, 193–201 (English edition).

Lukyanetz, E. A., Piper, T. P., Dolphin, A. C., and Sihra, T. S. (1996). Interaction between calcium channels and calcineurin in NG 108–15 cells. *J. Physiol. (London),* **494P**, 79P-80P.

Lynch, G. S., Dunwiddie, T., and Gribkoff, V. (1977). Heterosynaptic depression: a postsynaptic correlate of long-term potentiation. *Nature,* **266**, 737–9.

Magee, J. C., Avery, R. B., Christie, B. R., and Johnston, D. F. (1996). Dihydropyridine-sensitive, voltage-gated Ca^{2+} channels contribute to the resting intracellular Ca^{2+} concentration of hippocampal CA1 pyramidal neurons. *J. Neurophysiol.,* **76**, 3460–70.

Mak, D. O. D. and Foskett, J. K. (1997). Single-channel kinetics, inactivation, and spatial distribution of inositol triphosphate (IP3) receptors in *Xenopus* oocyte nucleus. *J. Gen. Physiol.,* **109**, 571–87.

Malen, P. L. and Chapman, P. F. (1997). Nitric oxide facilitates long-term potentiation, but not long-term depression. *J. Neurosci.,* **17**, 2645–51

Malenka, R. C., Lancaster, B., and Zucker, R. S. (1992). Temporal limits on the rise in postsynaptic calcium required for the induction of long-term potentiation. *Neuron,* **9**, 121–8.

Malinow, R. and Mainen, Y. F. (1996). Long-term potentiation in the CA1 hippocampus. *Science,* **271**, 1604–6.

Malinow, R., Liao, D., and Hessler, N. (1995). Postsynaptically silent synapses in CA1 hippocampus. In *Abstr. 4th IBRO World Congr. Neurosci.,* Kyoto, S4. 2.

Margaroli, A., Ting, A., Wendland, B., Bergamaschi, A., Villa, A., Tsien, R., *et al.* (1995). Presynaptic component of long-term potentiation visualized at individual hippocampal synapses. *Science,* **268**, 1624–8.

Martinez-Serrano, A., Vitorica, J., and Satrustegui, J. (1988). Cytosolic free calcium levels increase with age in rat brain synaptosomes. *Neurosci. Lett.,* **88**, 336–42.

Martinez-Serrano, A., Blanco, P., and Satrustegui, J. (1992). Calcium binding to the cytosol and calcium extrusion mechanisms in intact synaptosomes and their alteration with ageing. *J. Biol. Chem.,* **267**, 4672–9.

Masse, T. and Kelly, P. T. (1997). Overexpression of Ca^{2+}/calmodulin-dependent protein kinase II in PC12 cells alters cell growth, morphology, and nerve growth factor-induced differentiation. *J. Neurosci.,* **17**, 924–31.

Masuda-Nakagawa, L. M., Beck, K., and Chiquet, M. (1988). Identification of molecules in leech extracellular matrix that promote neurite outgrowth. *Proc. Royal Soc. London B.,* **235**, 247–57.

Masuda-Nakagawa, L. M., Muller, K. J., and Nicholls, J. G. (1990). Accumulation of laminin and microglial cells at sites of injury and regeneration in the central nervous system of the leech. *Proc. Royal Soc. London B.,* **241**, 201–6.

Mathie, A. and Richards, C. D. (1997). Calcium signalling in rat cortical neurones and glia in culture following activation of group I metabotropic glutamate receptors (μGluRs). *J. Physiol. (London),* **499P**, 18P-19P.

Mauelshagen, J., Parker, G. R., and Carew, T. J. (1996). Dynamics of induction and expression of long-term synaptic facilitation in Aplysia. *J. Neurosci.,* **16**, 7099–108.

McMahon, L. L. and Kauer, J. A. (1997) Hippocampal interneurons express a novel form of synaptic plasticity. *Neuron,* **19**, 295–305.

Mehta, S., Hsu, L., Jeng, A. Y., and Chen, K. Y. (1993). Neurite outgrowth and protein phosphorylation in chick embryonic sensory ganglia induced by a brief exposure to 12–*O*-tetradecanoylphorbol 13-acetate. *J. Neurochem.,* **60**, 972–81.

Michaelis, M. (1994). Ion transport systems and Ca^{2+} regulation in aging neurons. *Ann. New York Acad. Sci.,* **747**, 407–18.

Michaelis, M. L., Bigelow, D. J., Schöneich, C., Williams, T. D., Ramonda, L., Yin, D., *et al.* (1996). Decreased plasma membrane calcium transport activity in aging brain. *Life Sci.,* **59**, 405–12.

Michel, P. P. and Agid, Y. (1996). Chronic activation of the cyclic AMP signalling pathway promotes developmental and long-term survival of mesencephalic dopaminergic neurons. *J. Neurochem.,* **67**, 1633–42.

Miller, D. R., Lee, G. V., and Maness, P. F. (1993). Increased neurite outgrowth induced by inhibition of protein tyrosine kinase activity in PC12 pheochromocytoma cells. *J. Neurochem.,* **60**, 2134–44.

Miller, L. D. R., Petrozzino, J. J., Golarai, G., and Connor, J. A. (1996). Ca^{2+} release from untyracellular stores induced by afferent stimulation of CA3 pyramidal neurons in hippocampal slices. *J. Neurophysiol.,* **76**, 554–62.

Mione, M. C. and Parnavelas, J. G. (1994). How do developing cortical neurones know where to go? *Trends Neurosci.,* **11**, 443–5.

Mironov, S. L. and Lux, H. D. (1991). Calmodulin antagonists and protein phosphatase inhibitor okadaic acid fasten the 'run-up' of high-voltage activated calcium current in rat hippocampal neurones. *Neurosci. Lett.,* **133**, 175–8.

Monteith, G. R. and Roufogalis, B. D. (1995). The plasma membrane calcium pump—a physiological perspective on its regulation. *Cell Calcium,* **18**, 459–70.

Moorman, S. J. and Hume, R. I. (1993). ω-Conotoxin prevents myelin-evoked growth cone collapse in neonatal rat locus coeruleus neurons in vitro. *J. Neurosci.,* **13**, 4727–36.

Morris, S. A. and Bilezikian, J. P. (1986). Modification of adenylate cyclase complex during differentiation of cultured myoblasts. *J. Cell. Physiol.,* **127**, 28–38.

Mourre, C., Cervera, P., and Lazdunski, M. (1987). Autoradiographic analysis in rat brain of the postnatal ontogeny of voltage-dependent Na^{+} channels, Ca^{2+}-dependent K^{+} channels and slow Ca^{++} channels identified as receptors for tetrodotoxin, apamin and (–)-desmethoxyverapamil. *Brain Res.,* **417**, 21–32.

Mulkey, R. M. and Malenka, R. C. (1992). Mechanisms underlying induction of homosynaptic long-term depression in area CA1 of the hippocampus. *Neuron,* **9**, 967–75.

Mulkey, R. M. and Zucker, R. S. (1992). Posttetanic potentiation at the crayfish neuromuscular junction is dependent on both intracellular calcium and sodium ion accumulation. *J. Neurosci.,* **12**, 4327–36.

Mulkey, R. M., Herron, C. E., and Malenka, R. C. (1993). An essential role for protein phosphatases in hippocampal long-term depression. *Science,* **261**, 1051–55.

Muller, W. and Connor, J. A. (1991). Dendritic spines as individual neuronal compartments for synaptic Ca^{2+} responses. *Nature,* **354**, 73–6.

Murchison, D. and Griffith, W. H. (1995). Low-voltage activated calcium currents increase in basal forebrain neurons from aged rats. *J. Neurophysiol.,* **74**, 876–87.

Murchison, D. and Griffith, W. H. (1996). High-voltage-activated calcium currents in basal forebrain neurons during aging. *J. Neurophysiol.,* **76**, 158–74.

Mynlieff, M. and Beam, K. G. (1992). Developmental expression of voltage-dependent calcium currents in identified mouse motoneurons. *Dev. Biol.,* **152**, 407–10.

Nelson, Th. J., Collin, C., and Alkon, D. (1990). Isolation of a G protein that is modified by learning and reduces potassium currents in *Hermissenda. Science,* **247**, 1479–83.

Neveu, D. and Zucker, R. S. (1996*a*). Long-lasting potentiation and depression without presynaptic activity. *J. Neurophysiol.,* **75**, 2157–60.

Neveu, D. and Zucker, R. S. (1996*b*). Postsynaptic levels of $[Ca^{2+}]_i$ needed to trigger LTD and LTP. *Neuron,* **16**, 619–29.

Newman, E. A. and Zahs, K. R. (1997). Calcium waves in retinal glial cells. *Science,* **275**, 844–7.

Newman, E. A., Framback, D. A., and Odette, L. L. (1984). Control of extracellular potassium levels by retinal glial cells K siphoning. *Science,* **225**, 1174–5.

Norenberg, M. D. and Martinez-Hernandez, A. (1979). Fine structural localizations of glutamine synthetase in astrocytes of rat brain. *Brain Res.,* **161**, 303–10.

Nuijtinck, R. R. H., Baker, R. E., Ter Gast, E., Struik, M. L., and Mud, M. T. (1997). Glutamate dependent dendritic outgrowth in developing neuronal networks of rat hippocampal cells *in vitro. Int. J. Dev. Neurosci.,* **15**, 55–60.

Obrietan, K. and Van den Pol A. N. (1996). Growth cone calcium elevation by GABA. *J. Comp. Neurol.,* **372**, 167–75.

O'Dell, T. J. and Alger, B. E. (1991). Single calcium channels in rat and guinea-pig hippocampal neurones. *J. Physiol. (London),* **436**, 7739–76.

Ogura, A., Miyamoto, M., and Kudo, Y. (1988). Neuronal death in vitro: parallelism between survivability of hippocampal neurones and sustained elevation of cytosolic Ca^{++} after exposure to glutamate receptor agonist. *Exp. Brain Res.,* **73**, 447–59.

Orrenius, S., Ancarcrona, M., and Nicotera, P. (1996). Mechanisms of calcium-related cell death. In: *Advances in neurology, Vol. 71, Cellular and molecular mechanisms of ischemic brain damage.* (ed. B. K. Siesjö and T. Wieloch), pp. 138–51. Lippincott-Raven, Philadelphia.

Osaka, T. and Joyner, R. W. (1992). Developmental changes in the β-adrenergic modulation in calcium currents in rabbit ventricular cells. *Circ. Res.,* **70**, 104–15.

Papazafiri, P., Padini, P., Meldolesi, J., and Yamaguchi, T. (1995). Ageing affects cytosolic Ca^{2+} binding proteins and synaptic markers in the retina but not in cerebral cortex neurons of the rat. *Neurosci. Lett.,* **186**, 65–8.

Parri, H. R. and Lansman, J. B. (1996). Multiple components of Ca^{2+} channel facilitation in cerebellar granule cells: expression of facilitation during development in culture. *J. Neurosci.,* **16**, 4890–902.

Perkel, D. J., Petrozzino, J. J., Nicoll, R. A., and Connor, J. A. (1993). The role of Ca^{2+} entry via synaptically activated NMDA receptors in the induction of long-term potentiation. *Neuron,* **11**, 817–23.

Petersen, O. H. (1996*a*). Can Ca^{2+} be released from secretary granules or synaptic vesicles? *Trends Neurosci.,* **19**, 411–13.

Petersen, O. H. (1996*b*). New aspects of cytosolic calcium signalling. *News Physiol. Sci.,* **11**, 13–17.

Pitler, T. A. and Landfield, P. W. (1990). Aging-related prolongation of calcium spike duration in rat hippocampal slice neurons. *Brain Res.,* **508**, 1–6.

Porter, J. T. and McCarthy, K. D. (1995). Adenosine receptors modulate $[Ca^{2+}]_i$ in hippocampal astrocytes in situ. *J. Neurochem.,* **65**, 1515–23.

Pugh, P. C. and Berg, D. K. (1994). Neuronal acetylcholine receptors that bind α-bungarotoxin mediate neurite retraction in a calcium dependent manner. *J. Neurosci.,* **14**, 889–96.

Qian, X., Davis, A. A., Goderie, S. K., and Temple, S. (1997). FGF2 concentration regulates the generation of neurons and glia from multipotent cortical stem cells. *Neuron,* **18**, 81–93.

Regehr, W. G., Delaney, K. R., and Tank, D. W. (1994). The role of presynaptic calcium in short-term enhancement at the hippocampal mossy fiber synapse. *J. Neurosci.,* **14**, 523–37.

Rehder, V. and Kater, S. B. (1992). Regulation of neuronal growth cone filopodia by intracellular calcium. *J. Neurosci.,* **12**, 3175–86.

Rehder, V., Jensen, J. R., and Kater, S. B. (1992). The initial stages of neural regeneration are dependent upon intracellular calcium levels. *Neuroscience,* **51**, 565–74.

Reuter, H., Bouron, A., Neuhaus, R., Becker, C., and Reber, B. F. X. (1992). Inhibition of protein kinases in rat pheochromocytoma (PC12) cells promotes morphological differentiation and down-regulates ion channel expression. *Proc. Royal Soc. London B.,* **249**, 211–16.

Reyes, M. and Stanton, P. K. (1996). Induction of hippocampal long-term depression requires release of Ca^{2+} from separate presynaptic and postsynaptic intracellular stores. *J. Neurosci.,* **16**, 5951–60.

Reynolds, J. N. and Carlen, P. L. K. (1989). Diminished calcium currents in aged hippocampal dentate gyrus granule neurons. *Brain Res.,* **479**, 384–90.

Riedel, G. and Reymann, K. G. (1996). Metabotropic glutamate receptors in hippocampal long-term potentiation and learning and memory. *Acta Physiol. Scand.,* **157**, 1–19.

Ritchie, J. M. (1992). Voltage-gated ion channels in Schwann cells and glia. *Trends Neurosci.,* **15**, 345–51.

Rossi, P., D'Angelo, E., Magistretti, J., Toselli, M., and Taglietti, V. (1994). Age-dependent expression of high-voltage activated calcium currents during cerebellar granule cell development *in situ*. *Pfluegers Arch.,* **429**, 107–16.

Rossier, M. F., Burnay, M. M., Brandenburger, Y., Cherradi, N., Vallotton, M. B., and Capponi, A. M. (1996). Sources and sites of action of calcium in the regulation of aldosterone biosynthesis. *Endocrin. Res.,* **22**, 579–88.

Rusanescu, G., Qi, H., Thomas, S., Brugge, J., and Halegoua, S. (1995). Calcium influx induces neurite growth through a Src-Ras signalling cassette. *Neuron,* **15**, 1415–25.

Salin, P. A., Malenka, R. C., and Nicoll, R. A. (1996). Cyclic AMP mediates a presynaptic form of LTP at cerebellar parallel fiber synapses. *Neuron,* **16**, 797–803.

Sanchez-Vives, M. V. and Gallego, R. (1993). Effects of axotomy or target atrophy on membrane properties of rat sympathetic ganglion cells. *J. Physiol. (London),* **471**, 801–15.

Sanchez-Vives, M. V., Valdeolmillos, M., Martinez, S., and Gallego, R. (1994). Axotomy-induced changes in Ca^{2+} homeostasis in rat sympathetic ganglion cells. *Eur. J. Neurosci.,* **6**, 9–17.

Santella, L. (1996). The cell nucleus: an Eldorado to future calcium research? *J. Membr. Biol.,* **153**, 83–92.

Santi, C. M., Darszon, A., and Hernandez-Cruz, A. (1996). Dihydropyridine-sensitive T-type Ca^{2+} current is the main Ca^{2+} current carrier in mouse primary spermatocytes. *Am. J. Physiol. Cell Physiol.,* **271**, C1583-93.

Satrustegui, J., Villalba, M., Pereira, R., Bogonez, E., and Martinez-Serrano, A. (1996). Cytosolic and mitochondrial calcium in synaptosomes during aging. *Life Sci.,* **59**, 429–34.

Schiegg, A., Gerstner, W., Ritz, R., and Van Hemmen, J. L. (1995). Intracellular Ca^{2+} stores can account for the time course of LTP induction. A model of Ca^{2+} dynamics in dendritic spines. *J. Neurophysiol.,* **74**, 1046–55.

Schmid, S. and Guenther, E. (1996). Developmental regulation of voltage-activated Na^{+} and Ca^{++} currents in rat retinal ganglion cells. *NeuroReport,* **7**, 677–81.

Scholz, K. P. and Miller, R. J. (1995) Developmental changes in presynaptic calcium channels coupled to glutamate release in cultured rat hippocampal neurons. *J. Neurosci.,* **15**, 4612–17.

Scholz, K. P. and Miller, R. J. (1996). Presynaptic inhibition at excitatory hippocampal synapses: development and role of presynaptic Ca^{++} channels. *J. Neurophysiol.,* **76**, 39–46.

Schwartz, A., Palti, Y., and Meiri, H. (1990). Structural and developmental differences between three types of Na channels in dorsal root ganglion cells of newborn rats. *J. Membrane Biol.,* **116**, 117–28.

Schwartz, K. T. (1993). Modulation of Ca^{2+} channels by protein kinase C in rat central and peripheral neurons: disruption of G-protein mediated inhibition. *Neuron,* **11**, 305–20.

Shimachara, T., Melliti, K., and Bournaud, R. (1996). Voltage-dependent Ca^{2+} transients in Purkinje cells from mouse cerebellum. In: *Annual Meeting of Soc. for Exp. Biol.,* University of Lancaster, Animal and Animal/Cell Abstracts, p. 10.

Shitaka, Y., Matsuki, N., Saito, H., and Katsuki, H. (1996). Basic fibroblast growth factor increases functional L-type Ca^{++} channels in fetal rat hippocampal neurons: implications for neurite morphogenesis in vitro. *J. Neurosci.,* **16**, 6476–89.

Shmigol, A. V. and Kostyuk, E. P. (1995). Mechanisms responsible for calcium signal formation in murine primary sensory neurons: their impairment by experimental diabetes. *Neurophysiology (Kiev),* **27**, 261–9 (English edition).

Shmigol, A., Kostyuk, P., and Verkhratsky, A. (1995*a*). Dual action of thapsigargin on calcium mobilization in sensory neurons: inhibition of Ca^{2+} uptake by caffeine-sensitive pools and blockade of plasmalemmal Ca^{2+} channels. *Neuroscience,* **65**, 1109–18.

Shmigol, A., Kostyuk, P., and Verkhratsky, A. (1995*b*). Role of caffeine-sensitive Ca^{2+} stores in Ca^{2+} signal termination in adult mouse DRG neurons. *NeuroReport,* **5**, 2073–76.

Siegelbaum, S. A., Belardetti, F., Camardo, J. S., and Shuster, M. J. (1986). Modulation of the serotonin-sensitive potassium channels in *Aplysia* sensory neuron cell body and growth cone. *J. Exp. Biol.,* **124**, 287–306.

Siman, R., Bozyczko-Coyne, D., Savage, M. J., and Roberts-Lewis, J. M. (1996). The calcium-activated protease calpain I and ischemia-induced neurodegeneration. In: *Advances in Neurology, Vol. 71, Cellular and molecular mechanisms of ischemic brain damage.* (ed. B. K. Siesjö and T. Wieloch), pp. 167–75. Lippincott-Raven, Philadelphia.

Smith, R. G., Alexianu, M. E., Crawford, G, *et al.* (1994). Cytotoxicity of immunoglobulins from amyotropic lateral sclerosis patients on a hybrid motoneuron line. *Proc. Natl. Acad. Sci. USA,* **91**, 3393–7.

Snyder, D. L., Johnson, M. D., Aloyo, V., Eskin, B., and Roberts, J. (1995). Age-related changes in cardiac norepinephrin release: role of calcium movement. *J. Gerontol. (A),* **50A**, B358-B367.

Snyder, S. H. (1992). Nitric oxide: first in a new class of neurotransmitters. *Science,* **257**, 494–6.

Soeda, H., Tatsumi, H., and Katayama, Y. (1997) Neurotransmitter release from growth cones of rat dorsal root ganglion neurons in culture. *Neuroscience,* **77**, 1187–99.

Solem, N., McMahon, T., and Messing, R. O. (1995). Depolarization-induced neurite outgrowth in PC12 cells requires permissive, low level NGF receptor stimulation and activation of calcium/calmodulin-dependent protein kinase. *J. Neurosci.,* **15**, 5966–75.

Song, D.-K., Malstrom, T., Kater, S. B., and Mykles, D. L. (1994). Calpain inhibitors block Ca^{2+}-induced suppression of neurite outgrowth in isolated hippocampal pyramidal neurons. *J. Neurosci. Res.,* **39**, 474–81.

Sontheimer, H. (1994). Voltage-dependent ion channels in glial cells. *Glia,* **11**, 156–72.

Spitzer, N. C. (1991). A developmental handshake: neuronal control of ionic currents and their control of neuronal differentiation. *J. Neurobiol.,* **22**, 659–73.

Spitzer, N. C. (1994). Spontaneous Ca^{2+} spikes and waves in embryonic neurons: signalling systems for differentiation. *TINS,* **17**, 115–8.

Spitzer, N. C., Gu, X., and Olson, E. (1992). Calcium currents in embryonic nerve and muscle: triggers for differentiation. In *Advances in the innervation of the gastrointestinal tract,* (ed. G. E. Holle *et al.*), pp. 49–60. Elsevier.

Spitzer, N. C., Olson, E., and Gu, X. (1995). Spontaneous calcium transients regulate neuronal plasticity in developing neurons. *J. Neurobiol.,* **26**, 316–24.

Stanton, P. K. and Sejnowski, T. J. (1989). Associative long-term depression in the hippocampus induced by Hebbian covariance. *Nature,* **229**, 215–18.

Starikova, A. M., Chvanov, M. A., and Pogorelaya, N. Ch. (1997). Nifedipine-dependent changes in morphological differentiation and cytosolic calcium in rat pheochromocytoma cells. *Neurophysiology (Kiev),***29**, 374–5 (English edition).

Starikova, A. M., Chvanov, M. A., Pororelaya, N. Ch. and Kostyuk, P. G. (1998). Nifedipine induced morphological differentiation of rat pheochromocytoma cells. *Neuroscience,* **86**, in press.

Stoppini, L., Buchs, P.-A., and Muller, D. (1993). Lesion-induced neurite sprouting and synaptic formation in hippocampal organotypic cultures. *Neuroscience,* **57**, 985–94.

Suffel, J. L., Williams, E. J., Mason, I. J., Walsh, F. S., and Doherty, P. (1997). Expression of a dominant negative FGF receptor inhibits axonal growth and FGF receptor phosphorylation stimulated by CAMs. *Neuron,* **18**, 231–42.

Sun, X., Podratz, J. L., Gill, J. S., and Windebank, A. J. (1995). Action of extracellular calcium on suramin-induced inhibition of neurite outgrowth of cultured dorsal root ganglia. *J. Neurochem.,* **64**, Suppl., S26.

Svichar, N., Shmigol, A., Verkhratsky, A., and Kostyuk, P. (1997*a*). $InsP_3$-induced Ca^{2+} release in dorsal root ganglion neurones. *Neurosci. Lett.,* **227**, 107–10.

Svichar, N., Shmigol, A., Verkhratsky, A., and Kostyuk, P. (1997*b*). ATP induces Ca^{2+} release from IP_3-sensitive Ca^{2+} stores exclusively in large DRG neurons. *NeuroReport,* **8**, 1555–9.

Sweatt, J. D. and Kandel, E. R. (1989). Persistent and transcriptionally-dependent increase in protein phosphorylation in long-term facilitation of *Aplysia* sensory neurons. *Nature,* **339**, 51–4.

Takei, K., Stukenbrok, H., Metcalf, A., Mignery, G. A., Sudhof, T. C., Vople, P., *et al.* (1992). Ca^{2+} stores in Purkinje neurons: endoplasmic reticulum subcompartments demonstrated by the heterogeneous distribution of the $InsP_3$ receptor, Ca^{2+}-ATPase, and calsequestrin. *J. Neurosci.,* **12**, 489–505.

Takeichi, M. (1987). Cadherins: a molecular family essential for selective cell-cell adhesion in animal morphogenesis. *Trends Genet.,* **3**, 213–17.

Tanaka, S. and Koike, T. (1995). Up-regulation of L-type Ca^{2+} channel associated with the development of elevated K^+-mediated survival of superior cervical ganglion cells in vitro. *Dev. Biol.,* **168**, 166–78.

Tanaka, T., Saito, H., and Matsuki, N. (1997). Inhibition of $GABA_A$ synaptic responses by brain-derived neurotrophic factor (BDNF) in rat hippocampus. *J. Neurosci.,* **17**, 2959–66.

Tang, Y.-G. and Zucker, R. S. (1997). Mitochondrial involvement in posttetanic potentiation of synaptic transmission. *Neuron,* **18**, 483–91.

Tarasenko, A. N., Kostyuk, P. G., Eremin, A. V., and Isaev, D. S. (1997). Two types of low-voltage-activated Ca^{2+} channel in neurones of rat laterodorsal thalamic nucleus. *J. Physiol. (London),* **499**, 77–86.

Tarasenko, A. N., Isaev, D. S., Eremin, A. V. and Kostyuk, P. G. (1998). Developmental changes in expression of low-voltage-operated Ca^{2+} channels in rat visual cortical neurones. *J. Physiol. (London).* **508**, in press.

Teng, K. K. and Greene, L. A. (1993). Depolarization maintains neurites and priming of PC12 cells after nerve growth factor withdrawal. *J. Neurosci.,* **13**, 3124–35.

Teyler, T., Cavis, I., Coussens, C., DiScenna, P., Grover, L., Lee, Y. P., *et al.* (1994). Multideterminant role of calcium in hippocampal synaptic plasticity. *Hippocampus,* **4**, 623–34.

Thibault, O. and Landfield, P. W. (1996). Increase in single L-type calcium channels in hippocampal neurons during aging. *Science,* **272**, 1017–20.

Thompson, S. M. and Wong, R. K. S. (1991). Development of calcium current subtypes in isolated rat hippocampal pyramidal cells. *J. Physiol. (London),* **434**, 671–89.

Torii, N., Kamishita, T., Otsu, Y., and Tsumoto, T. (1995). An inhibitor for calcineurin, FK506, blocks induction of long-term depression in rat visual cortex. *Neurosci. Lett.*, **185**, 1–4.

Trump, B. F. and Berezesky, I. K. (1995). Calcium-mediated cell injury and cell death. *FASEB J.*, **9**, 219–28.

Trump, B. F. and Berezesky, I. K. (1996). The role of altered $[Ca^{2+}]_i$ regulation in apoptosis, oncosis, and necrosis. *Biochem. Biophys. Acta*, **1313**, 173–8.

Tsai, H., Duckles, S. P., and Buchholz, J. (1995). Rat tail artery norepinephrine release: age and effect of mitochondrial blockade. *Neurobiol. Aging*, **16**, 773–7.

Tsakiridou, E., Bertollini, L., De Curtis, M., Avazini, G., and Pape, H.-C. (1995). Selective increase in T-type calcium conductance of reticular thalamic neurons in a rat model of absence epilepsy. *J. Neurosci.*, **15**, 3110–7.

Tse, F. W., Tse, A., Hille, B., Horstmann, H., and Almers, W. (1997). Local Ca^{2+} release from internal stores controls exocytosis in pituitary gonadotrophs. *Neuron*, **18**, 121–32.

Tsintsadze, T., Lozovaya, N., Klishin, A., and Krishtal, O. (1996). NMDA receptor-mediated synapses between CA1 neurones: activation by ischemia. *NeuroReport*, **7**, 2679–82.

Venance, L., Stella, N., Glowinski, J., and Giaume, C. (1997). Mechanism involved in initiation and propagation of receptor-induced intercellular calcium signalling in cultured rat astrocytes. *J. Neurosci.*, **17**, 1981–92.

Verderio, C., Coco, S., Fumagalli, G., and Matteoli, M. (1994) Spatial changes in calcium signalling during the establishment of neuronal polarity and synaptogenesis. *J. Cell Biol.*, **126**, 1527–36.

Verhage, M., Chijsen, W. E. J. M., and Lopes da Silva, F. H. (1994). Presynaptic plasticity: the regulation of Ca^{++}-dependent transmitter release. *Progr. Neurobiol.*, **42**, 539–74.

Verkhratsky, A., Shmigol, A., Kirischuk, S., Pronchuk, N., and Kostyuk, P. (1994). Age-dependent changes in calcium currents and calcium homeostasis in mammalian neurons. *Ann. New York Acad. Sci.*, **747**, 365–81.

Vernadakis, A. (1996). Glia-neuron intercommunications and synaptic plasticity. *Progr. Neurobiol.*, **49**, 185–214.

Vernadakis, A. and Kentroti, S. (1994). Glial cells derived from aged mouse brain in culture display both mature and immature astrocyte phenotypes. *J. Neurosci.*, **38**, 451–8.

Veselovsky, N. S. and Fomina, A. F. (1986). Sodium and calcium channels in the somatic membrane of artificially differentiated neuroblastoma cells. *Neurophysiology (Kiev)*, **18**, 154–8 (English edition).

Veselovsky, N. S., Pogorelaya, N. Kh., and Fomina, A. F. (1984). Calcium currents in differentiated cells of mouse neuroblastoma. *Neurophysiology (Kiev)*, **16**, 419–22 (English edition).

Veselovsky, N. S., Fedulova, S. A., and Kostyuk, P. G. (1986). Changes in ionic mechanisms of electrical excitability of the somatic membrane of rat's dorsal root ganglion neurons during ontogenesis. Relationship between calcium channels functioning and intracellular metabolism. *Neurophysiology (Kiev),* **18**, 587–90 (English edition).

Villalba, M., Bockaert, J., and Jopurnot, L. (1997). Pituitary adenylate cyclase-activating polypeptide (PACAP-38) protects cerebellar granule neurons from apoptosis by activating the mitogen-activated protein kinase (MAP kinase) pathway. *J. Neurosci.,* **17**, 83–90.

Vincent, A. and Drachman, D. B. (1996). Amyotrophic lateral sclerosis and antibodies to voltage-gated calcium channels—new doubts. *Ann. Neurol.,* **40**, 691–3.

Villa, A., Podini, P., Panzeri, M. C., Racchetti, G., and Meldolesi, J. (1994). Cytosolic Ca^{2+} binding proteins during rat brain ageing: loss of calbindin and calretinin in the hippocampus, with no change in the cerebellum. *Eur. J. Neurosci.,* **6**, 1491–9.

Vlassara, H., Bucala, L. and Striker, L. (1994). Biology of disease. Pathogenic effects of advanced glycosylation: biochemical, biologic, and clinical implications for diabetes and aging. *Lab. Invest.*, **70**, 138–51.

Voronin, L. L. (1993). On the quantal analysis of hippocampal long-term potentiation and related phenomena of synaptic plasticity. *Neuroscience,* **56**, 275–304.

Vyatchenko-Karpinskii, S. V., Pogorelaya, N. Kh., Magura, I. S., Rozhmanova, O. M., Kvasyuk, V. I., and Mikhailopulo, I. A. (1995*a*). α-Interferon- and oligoadenylate-induced morphological differentiation and modulation of the ion channels in neuroblastoma cells. *Neurophysiology (Kiev),* **27**, 156–63 (English edition).

Vyatchenko-Karpinskii, S. V., Pogorelaya, N. Ch., Tokhtuev, A. E., and Sedova, M. B. (1995*b*). Effect of verapamil on morphological differentiation and low-threshold calcium current of murine neuroblastoma cells. *Neurophysiology (Kiev),* **27**, 208–13 (English edition).

Wang, J.-H. and Stelzer, A. (1994). Inhibition of phosphatase 2B prevents expression of hippocampal long-term potentiation. *NeuroReport,* **5**, 2377–80.

Wang, J.-H. and Stelzer, A. (1996). Shared calcium signalling pathways in the induction of long-term potentiation and synaptic disinhibition in CA1 pyramidal cell dendrites. *J. Neurophysiol.,* **75**, 1687–702.

Wang, L., Bhattacharjee, A., Fu, L. A., and Li, M. (1996). Abnormally expressed low-voltage activated calcium channels in β-cells from NOD mice and a related clonal cell line. *Diabetes,* **45**, 1678–83.

Wang, Y., Rowan, M. J., and Anwyl, R. (1996) Evidence that long-term depression induction in the rat hippocampus in vitro requires Ca^{2+} influx via Ni^{2+}-sensitive Ca^{2+} channels and Ca^{2+} release from intracellular stores. *J. Physiol. (London),* **495**, 50P.

Webb, B., Suarez, S. S., Heaton, M. B., and Walker, D. W. (1996). Cultured postnatal rat medial septal neurons respond to acute ethanol treatment and nerve growth factor by changing intracellular calcium levels. *Alcohol. Clin. Exp. Res.,* **20**, 1385–94.

Weisskopf, M. G. and Nicoll, R. A. (1995). Presynaptic changes during mossy fibre LTP revealed by NMDA receptor-mediated synaptic responses. *Nature,* **376**, 256–9.

Westenbroek, R. E., Hell, J., Warner, C., Dubel, S., Snutch, T., and Catterall, W. A. (1992). Biochemical properties and subcellular distribution of an N-type calcium channel α_1 subunit. *Neuron,* **9**, 1099–115.

Wildeling, W. C., Lodder, J. C., Kits, K. S., and Bulloch, A. G. M. (1995). Nerve growth factor (NGF) acutely enhances high-voltage activated calcium currents in molluscan neurons. *J. Neurophysiol.,* **74**, 2778–81.

Williams, D. K. and Cohan, C. S. (1995). Calcium transients in growth cones and axons of cultured *Helisoma* neurons in response to conditioning factors. *J. Neurobiol.,* **27**, 60–75.

Williams, E. J., Walsh, F. S., and Doherty, O. (1994). The production of arachidonic acid can account for calcium channel activation in the second messenger pathway underlying neurite outgrowth by NCAM, N-cadherin, and LI. *J. Neurochem.,* **62**, 1231–4.

Wind, T., Prehn, J. H. M., Peruche, B., and Krieglstein, J. (1997). Activation of ATP-sensitive potassium channels decreases neuronal injury caused by chemical hypoxia. *Brain Res.,* **751**, 295–9.

Winiewski, T. and Frangione, B. (1996). Molecular biology of brain aging and neurodegenerative disorders. *Acta Neurobiol. Exp.,* **56**, 267–79.

Xia, Z., Choi, E.-J., Storm, D. R., and Blazynski, C. (1995). Do the calmodulin-stimulated adenylyl cyclases play a role in neuroplasticity? *Behav. Brain Sci.,* **18**, 429–40.

Xiong, Z., Sperelakis, N., Noffsinger, A., and Fenoglio-Preiser, C. (1995). Potassium currents in rat colonic smooth muscle cells and changes during development and aging. *Pfluegers Arch.,* **430**, 563–72.

Xu, X. and Best, P. M. (1992). Postnatal changes in L-type calcium current density in rat atrial myocytes. *J. Physiol. (London),* **454, 657–72.**

Yamamoto, S., Tanaka, E., and Higashi, H. (1997). Mediation by intracellular calcium-dependent signals of hypoxic hyperpolarization in rat hippocampal CA1 neurons in vitro. *J. Neurophysiol.,* **77**, 386–92.

Yuasa, S., Kawamura, K., Kuwano, R., and Ono, K. (1996). Neuron-glia interrelations during migration of Purkinje cells in the mouse embryonic cerebellum. *Int. J. Dev. Neurosci.,* **14**, 429–38.

Zhang, C., Brandemihl, A., Lau, D., Lawton, A., and Oakley, B. (1997). BDNF is required for the normal development of taste neurons *in vivo*. *NeuroReport,* **8**, 1013–7.

Zheng, J. Q., Felder, M., Connor, J. A., and Poo, M.-M. (1994). Turning of nerve growth cones induced by neurotransmitters. *Nature,* **368**, 140–4.

Zimprich, F. and Bolsover, S. R. (1995). A higher density of L-type calcium channels at the tip of neuroblastoma growth cones in culture causes a gradient of Ca^{++} influx. *J. Physiol. (London),* **489P**, 14P.

Zimprich, F. and Bolsover, S. R. (1996). Calcium channels in neuroblastoma cell growth cones. *Eur. J. Neurosci.,* **8**, 467–75.

Zimprich, F., Gailey, M., and Bolsover, S. R. (1994). Biphasic effect of calcium on neurite outgrowth in neuroblastoma and cerebellar granule cells. *Dev. Brain Res.,* **80**, 7–12.

Zucker, R. S. (1994). Calcium and short-term synaptic plasticity. *Netherlands J. Zool.,* **44**, 495–512.

Index